# Developing Research in Primary Care

Edited by

Mike Saks

Martin Williams

and

Beverley Hancock

Foreword by

Mike Pringle

Radcliffe Medical Press

Radcliffe Medical Press Ltd
18 Marcham Road, Abingdon, Oxon OX14 1AA

British Library Cataloguing in Publication Data

A catalogue record for this book is available from the British Library.

ISBN 1 85775 397 6

Typeset by Advance Typesetting Ltd, Oxfordshire
Printed and bound by TJ International Ltd, Padstow, Cornwall

# Contents

# Foreword

Research into primary care is underdeveloped, not just amongst general practitioners but also nurses and other health professionals. Primary care cannot be expected to move from the twilight into the spotlight without support. The welcome access for general practices and community trusts to Culyer research and development funding has started to redress the resource inequality between primary and secondary care. However, the greatest shortage has been in research skills, as those involved have not routinely been expected to undertake research in their training and, for many, research skills appear foreign and demanding.

The recognition of these realities led Trent Regional Health Authority – now the Trent Regional Office of the NHS Executive – to support the Trent Focus for the Promotion of Research and Development in Primary Health Care from 1995 onwards. The Focus has existed primarily to enhance the research skills of those working in primary care on a regional basis. It does this through offering education and support to those interested in research; buying specific research advice for those undertaking research; supporting research clubs; running a collaborating research practices scheme and funding designated research practices which undertake original research.

Out of this work recognition emerged that some research issues came up time and again, and that the standard reference works do not cover them satisfactorily. Thus the idea for this series was born. These volumes synthesise current wisdom on how to start successfully in primary care research. They are not intended to provide definitive texts, nor to be used as the only source of knowledge. They will, however, cover most of the issues that a nascent researcher will encounter, and will inspire many to try their hand.

For the truth is this: research can be wonderfully stimulating, enriching our daily clinical work and helping to improve care for future generations. However, like most areas of human activity, it is only worth doing if it is done well – and that requires skills, support, advice, insight and perseverance. Those who read and use these volumes will stand a better chance of doing good research, and should obtain real pleasure from it.

Professor Mike Pringle
Chairman
RCGP
*October 1999*

# Volume editors

**Professor Mike Saks**
Dean of Faculty of Health and
     Community Studies
De Montfort University, Leicester

**Martin Williams**
Trent Focus Local Coordinator
De Montfort University

**Beverley Hancock**
Trent Focus Local Coordinator
Division of General Practice, University
     of Nottingham

# List of contributors

**Antony John Arthur**
Research Associate in Nursing
Department of Epidemiology and
    Public Health, University of Leicester

**Dr Richard Baker**
Director of Clinical Governance Research
    and Development Unit
Department of General Practice
    and Primary Care,
    University of Leicester

**Linda East**
Lecturer
School of Nursing (Postgraduate
    Division), University of Nottingham

**Andy Farrington**
Lecturer in Mental Health Nursing
School of Nursing, University of
    Nottingham

**Vicky Hammersley**
Trent Focus Network Coordinator
Division of General Practice, University
    of Nottingham

**Dr Michael Hewitt**
Research Associate
Trent Institute for Health Services
    Research and Nottingham Community
    Health NHS Trust

**Amanda Howe**
Senior Lecturer
Institute of General Practice and
    Primary Care, University of Sheffield

**Amanda Hunn**
Trent Focus Local Coordinator
Institute of General Practice and
    Primary Care, University
    of Sheffield

**Professor Nigel Mathers**
Director
Institute of General Practice and
    Primary Care, University
    of Sheffield

**Jane Schober**
Principal Lecturer
Department of Nursing and Midwifery,
    De Montfort University, Leicester

# Introduction

*Mike Saks*

The six chapters in this volume cover in a straightforward manner a number of facets of the research process relevant to those wishing actively to develop research in primary care. Whilst the significance of continuing to raise awareness of research in this area should by no means be downplayed, the task of actually undertaking such research is also extremely important at a time when evidence-based practice has become such a crucial feature of healthcare in Britain and many other Western societies. This is particularly accentuated in the field of primary care where research remains relatively underdeveloped, even though this is now rapidly beginning to change. This volume and others in the series will play their part in facilitating the necessary research shift in this field, as primary care becomes ever more central to the National Health Service agenda in this country.

The first chapter in this book by Anthony Arthur is a practical guide to starting a research project and, most importantly, to applying for the funding that is required for most serious research into primary care. As such, it not only provides an overview of a range of key aspects of the research process, but also helpfully highlights the wide span of sources of funding available for different forms of research in this area. This is complemented by a useful indication of the type of information that funding bodies are seeking in research proposals which should increase the chances of applicants achieving a successful outcome from their submissions. As with subsequent chapters in this volume, the chapter also includes active exercises for the reader to undertake to reinforce the main messages contained in the text.

The second chapter by Michael Hewitt provides further in-depth guidance on carrying out a literature review as a vital initial step in the research process in primary care. Aside from underlining the importance of conducting a review of already published work in the field of research concerned, this contribution provides help for readers interested in systematically conducting a literature search. This is seen to include the use of bibliographic tools in both their paper and electronic forms, the specific nature of which is informatively explored. The chapter also considers the skills required to review critically the existing literature base in particular areas. The acquisition and use of such skills is felt to be essential in highlighting the issues to be considered in the proposed research in primary care.

In the third chapter, Nigel Mathers, Amanda Howe and Amanda Hunn address the sensitive question of ethical considerations, which are integral to undertaking any form of research project. As they note, it is particularly critical for anyone embarking on research involving patients in the health sector in primary care. The chapter begins with a discussion of general ethical principles and their application to research. It then builds on this philosophical base, by pragmatically outlining the processes for obtaining informed consent and making applications for ethical approval through research ethics committees. The authors usefully adopt a challenging approach to this part of the volume by pro-actively inviting the reader to consider potential pitfalls in this field and how these may be overcome.

The fourth chapter by Linda East, Vicky Hammersley and Beverley Hancock moves on to focus specifically on health needs assessment, with the aim of providing the reader with an understanding of the main principles involved. In so doing, it sets out a number of different approaches to health needs assessment, highlights a range of methods for gathering associated data and considers the way in which such information may be interpreted and applied. This aspect of the research agenda again has particular applicability to practitioners in primary care, enabling due recognition to be given to the multifaceted group context in which individuals lead their lives in particular localities. The value of health needs assessment is that it has the potential to improve health in line with government policy at a time when there is great pressure to engage in sensitive prioritisation in allocating scarce resources in the National Health Service.

The next chapter by Jane Schober and Andy Farrington gives basic advice on presenting and disseminating research. Their chapter is centred on outlining the elements that comprise a written-up research project, including the various forms that this may take depending on purpose. In this regard, they particularly focus on the construction of research reports and research dissertations, emphasising the contribution that these can make to professional practice. This latter consideration includes a discussion of the range of channels for disseminating research – not least being publications and conferences – which the committed researcher will wish to pursue selectively. Importantly, they stress that research in primary care must not be seen as simply being conducted and diffused by isolated researchers, but through multidisciplinary collaboration.

In the final chapter by Richard Baker the implementation of research is discussed in a primary care context. As such, it covers the stage in the research process which typically follows on from the writing up of results. The chapter strives to help practitioners to be aware of where to find and how to appraise sources of research data, in which they are now greatly aided by the development of systematic reviews. It also examines the difficulties that can be involved in implementing research findings, as well as more positively considering the as yet incomplete evidence on the strategies that can lead to success in this respect. This is vital if primary care is to become more effective in the interprofessional teams that are increasingly involved in its delivery in an era in which there is growing support for evidence-based medicine.

Linking the development of the research process to the dissemination and implementation of soundly grounded research outcomes is critical if the loop between those who actively design and carry out research and those who have a responsibility to apply research findings in primary care and other contexts is to be effectively closed. The chapters in this volume are intended to make a practical and meaningful contribution to this agenda – not just for those directly starting research projects in this field, but also for primary care practitioners anxious to gain some general insight into how research is carried out and how it can be utilised in their work. In this respect, it is hoped that at least some of the readers of this volume will go on from this voyage of discovery of today to become the experienced researchers and systematic implementers of research in primary care of tomorrow.

# CHAPTER ONE

# Starting a research project and applying for funding

*Antony John Arthur*

## Introduction

The aims of this chapter are:

- to enable primary care staff to build research ideas into an application for funding from a greater understanding of the research process
- to increase awareness among primary care staff of the potential for obtaining funding for research activity
- to gain skills in recognising good and bad practice in writing a research proposal.

If a project is worth doing then it is probably worth convincing an interested organisation to fund it. There are no ways of guaranteeing funding but there are steps you can take to maximise your chances of success. Applying for research funding might sound like the starting point of the research process but applicants need to demonstrate a clear idea of what will happen at the end of the process in terms of outcomes (for example, modes of dissemination and practical implementation of results) in order to convince funding bodies that their money will be spent wisely.

In 1997 the Department of Health reported:

> 'The NHS Research and Development strategy aims to create a knowledge-based health service in which clinical, managerial and policy decisions are based on sound information about research findings and scientific developments.'

Health services research is valued highly because it provides information for evidence-based practice. Similarly, with increasing recognition that health services are inherently multidisciplinary, so research that evaluates those services should be carried out by all healthcare professions. It is a particularly good time for those in primary care to become active in research. Historically, research has predominantly been carried out in the acute sector, but with the shift towards a primary care-led NHS comes the need for the evaluation of primary care services and for research to inform practice.

## How to use this chapter

This chapter is intended to give those working in primary healthcare a starting point for applying for research funds. The first section takes the reader through the steps of the research process. The activities in this section are designed to get you to start putting together a research application that is worth funding. The second section looks at the context of funding for health services research in the UK and provides a framework to illustrate the main types of research funding available. The third section takes a typical research grant application form and breaks it down into the component parts to look at the sort of information and messages funding bodies and referees are looking for. This section can be used by the reader to draft out their research design into a grant proposal, and at the end of this section the reader is asked to critically appraise their draft application. The fourth section gives the reader some insights into the experience of applying and not always getting research funds. Jargon and terms used in the world of health services research are not always easily understood by those new to the game and a glossary is therefore included on p. 143. Finally, at the end of the chapter, beginning on p. 25, details of sources are given that the reader may find useful when considering applying for research funds.

For those new to research, obtaining funds to carry out projects or training may seem like a daunting task. A study of grant applications carried out in Wales suggests that research committees do not restrict awards to those with a track record, nor are they biased towards particular professional groups (Mead 1997). It is hoped that this chapter will encourage primary care staff to view funding as a necessary part of research activity and that the process of application for research funding can be a sound investment of time and reap long-term rewards.

# The research process

This section is designed to get you thinking about your research project. Most general textbooks on research methods will have an introductory chapter on the research process and the various stages of activity from first thoughts to utilising research-based evidence. The process outlined here is chronological and practical. In the real world of research this idealised process is far less straightforward: study designs are modified, research questions beg other lines of scientific enquiry and changes in the way health services are provided force different methods of sampling and approach.

Interspersed throughout this section is an example from a published paper (Singh *et al.* 1997) to demonstrate the way in which one piece of research appeared to deal with different parts of the research process. There are also eight activities that should not take up too much of your time but will get you to start firming up your own ideas into a research proposal.

## Research idea

If you have read this far, the chances are that you have already got some rough idea of a research project you might like to carry out. It may only be a hunch at this stage, or an area of interest that you would like to explore further. Ideas may come from a variety of sources: interesting patients, something you have read, conversations with others. Now is the time to brainstorm.

### Exercise 1

Write down the subject area(s) that have been nagging away at you for a while. Think about why they interest you and what was the trigger that made you interested in them in the first place. You are probably worried that your ideas are vague. Elegant research projects start with vague ideas and to move forward from this starting point involves getting something (however embryonic) down on paper.

---

**Box 1.1**    Example

The subject of interest is depression in elderly people, with a particular interest in alternative or additional forms of treatment. It has been noticed that regular exercise seems to have a positive effect on other groups (for example, patients following myocardial infarction) not only in terms of their physical health but also in terms of their mental health. This is the starting point – the research idea – could physical exercise help older people with depression?

---

## Trawling the literature

You will have got together a few keywords by now which is enough to do a literature search. A good librarian can help you with this and let you know what literature databases are available, which are most suitable for your area of interest, and whether there is any cost involved in carrying out the search. For guidance in undertaking this you may wish to contact your local health sciences or hospital library.

Do not rely on computerised databases alone and if you are aware of a good paper on the subject, check through the references to see what else you may need to get hold of. Your first attempt at a database search may result in turning up one publication in the last ten years, or 2000 references per year, bringing the system to a standstill. This is common and is an indication of the need to expand or refine your search rather than give up at the first hurdle.

Carrying out a literature search is not a trivial job but avoid the urge to track down every possible reference that is vaguely connected to your subject area. More recent articles are likely to summarise older work anyway. Allow yourself time to spend in a library to actually look at some of the references that you turn up. Some you will need photocopies of, but photocopying is not a substitute for reading. When you get down to some selective but serious reading, certain themes should start to emerge from the literature, and the gaps in the literature should soon appear giving you the background to your proposed study.

---

**Box 1.2**   Example

A number of keywords for this area of interest comes to mind. 'Depression', 'elderly' and 'exercise' are the most obvious. These are broad areas and most databases such as MEDLINE or BIDS will allow you to restrict your search to papers where your keyword is the main focus.

---

*Exercise 2*

List the most relevant keywords to your own area of interest sketched out in Exercise 1. In the example in Box 1.2 the keywords fall neatly under three headings: the problem ('depression'), the population ('elderly') and the potential intervention or solution ('exercise'). If you have a number of keywords it may help to group them under these or other types of headings. Not only will this ensure that time spent searching databases is used wisely, but it will also start to order your research ideas into a more manageable form.

## Research question

Having a clear research question is essential for a successful project. Funding bodies understand this and are unlikely to back an application based on vague aims. The research question should guide the project from this point on. If it is too ambitious you may have to modify it, but you should never throw it out without something to replace it. Interest in carrying out a study of the effectiveness of health promotion clinics is to be at the idea stage rather than having a researchable question. A research question should include the area of interest (for example, nurse-led health promotion clinics), the section of the population you might wish to investigate (for example, clinic attenders aged between 20 and 65 years) and the specific issue you are seeking to address in the study (for example, giving up smoking).

---

**Box 1.3** Example

Based on a literature review of (i) depression in the elderly, (ii) the effect of exercise on mental health and (iii) exercise and older people, the following conclusions can be drawn:

- Standard therapy for treatment of depression among older people is drug treatment, but many older people cannot comply with antidepressant medication because of side-effects.
- In studies of younger adults there is evidence to suggest that aerobic and resistance (weight) training can help mildly depressed patients.
- Modified resistance training appears to have higher compliance than aerobic exercise and is safer for older people who are at risk of injury from falls.

From this summary of the literature, a research question can be posed:

*Can weight training improve the quality of life in depressed older people?*

The research question clearly begs other questions:
What is meant by weight training?
How is quality of life measured?
How do we define depressed older people?
These questions need to be addressed as the study is designed.

---

*Exercise 3*

The following titles are taken from recent publications and either take the form of a research question or are answers to a research question:

Improving uptake of breast screening in multi-ethnic populations: a randomised controlled trial using practice reception staff to contact non-attenders (*British Medical Journal*)
A descriptive study of the readability of patient information leaflets designed by nurses (*Journal of Advanced Nursing*)
How common is medical training in palliative care? A postal survey of general practitioners (*British Journal of General Practice*).

To get yourself familiar with good research questions, have a look at a recent journal that publishes papers reporting original research. Pick out three titles and identify the following components: outcomes (for example, improved uptake in breast screening; readability of leaflets), interventions or potential causative agents (practice staff contacting non-attenders), populations (multi-ethnic populations, general practitioners) and study design (randomised controlled trial; postal survey).

Now have a go at putting your own research question together. It should include some (though not necessarily all) of the components mentioned above.

## Study design

Now comes the hard part. You will probably have already got a picture in your own mind of the kind of study you are hoping to carry out. The most important consideration in choosing an overall study design is that it should be feasible and appropriate to the subject of interest. If you are attempting to evaluate a new therapy/service and compare it with an existing therapy/service then a randomised controlled trial (RCT) is probably your best bet. For looking at levels of disability, or prevalence of different types of attitude to certain health behaviours or health services, a cross-sectional study is likely to be more appropriate. In order to understand links between exposures and diseases then, depending on time, money and the number of potential recruits to your study, a case–control or cohort study is probably the study design of choice. A good textbook on health services research methods will cover the differences and relative advantages and disadvantages of each type of study design.

---

**Box 1.4**    Example

The research question 'Can weight training improve the quality of life in depressed older people?' is attempting to evaluate an intervention (weight training), and an RCT was considered the most appropriate study design.

The problem of definition was addressed as follows:

*weight training*: a supervised exercise training regimen of resistance training of the large muscle groups (chosen for their importance in functional activities). A session lasting approximately 45 minutes took place three days a week for ten weeks.
*quality of life*: this was broken down into separate domains (depression, morale and physical functioning) with previously validated instruments used to measure each domain.
*depressed older people*: subjects aged 60 years and over who fulfilled a specified diagnostic criteria.

Design of the RCT: two volunteer databases were used and all those aged 60 years and over were sent a screening instrument for depression and those scoring over a specified score were contacted by phone to see if they (i) fulfilled the diagnostic criteria; (ii) were not ineligible on grounds of recent treatment with antidepressant medication, recent weight training exercise or suffering from unstable diseases; and (iii) agreed to take part in the study. These subjects were then invited to attend a local clinic for assessment and then randomised into either the intervention group (to undertake the ten-week resistance training) or the control group. Control subjects took part in an interactive health education programme to ensure that any improved outcomes in the intervention group was not the result of the increased social contact gained during the exercise. Outcomes were measured at the end of the ten-week period.

---

*Exercise 4*

From your research question decide how you are going to define your study group (in terms of age, sex, presence or absence of certain conditions, receiving or not receiving certain services, etc.) and the concepts you are interested in. Even the most straight-forward of concepts need definition. Take smoking for instance: do you include people who consider themselves ex-smokers? Those that smoke socially? People who smoke only cigars? Will you measure extent of smoking by average daily number of cigarettes? What if the number of cigarettes smoked in the week differs substantially from that smoked at the weekend?

Now try and sketch out your study design. If you are attempting a cross-sectional survey you might want to start making a list of the sort of data you want to collect and the type of questions you are going to be asking. If your study is longitudinal it is probably easiest to do this in diagrammatic form, especially if different groups of participants take different pathways (as in an RCT or in a study where the first stage is cross-sectional and a subsample of participants go on to a second stage).

## Applying for funds

At this point in the research process it is useful to start thinking about who is likely to pay for this type of research. This will depend on whether it is a local and/or national issue, and whether there is a suitable charity which funds research. It is also worth thinking about how much time and money the project is likely to cost. Research time in the form of staffing costs are usually the biggest part of any grant application, but service costs need to be included if, for example, you need to run extra clinics to assess participants in your study. Equipment is also expensive. Stationery and travel costs are easy to overlook but need to be budgeted for. The section 'Who funds research?' (p. 15) gives details of types of funding, major grant-making organisations and useful resources for finding an appropriate funding body.

*Exercise 5*

Write down three good reasons why you think your project should be funded. Be authoritative and confident! If you have reached this point in the activities set so far, then you obviously believe that you have a potentially valuable project on your hands. Use your keywords to think about potential sources of funding.

## Sampling

If your research question is well thought through, you should be able to state clearly your inclusion and exclusion criteria for the potential study. A suitable sampling frame will be needed and a decision made on whether to include all who satisfy the inclusion criteria or whether a sample should be taken. Most general practices and all health authorities have computerised registers. As a general rule, when taking a sample, random is best. If you have good reasons for taking a non-random sample, then those reasons will need to be stated when applying for funding and later on when writing up the study. The size of the sample you will need to take will depend on a number of factors: time and resources available, prevalence of the condition you are studying and likely response rate. If you want to undertake an RCT you will need to carry out a power calculation.

How you carry out a power calculation is one of the most frequently asked questions of statisticians working in health services research and you are advised to consult a statistician for this. It is a relatively simple procedure but if you get it wrong it will have the effect of carrying out a trial unnecessarily large, or one too small to be able to evaluate your intervention.

## Exercise 6

Try and estimate how many eligible participants there are for your study. If you work in general practice and your subjects are going to include men and women, and be between two specified ages, find out how many patients are registered who fall into this group. If you then want to look at a particular group with a particular condition (for example, those with non-insulin dependent diabetes), using your knowledge of the prevalence of the condition, calculate how many potentially eligible patients there will be in your study. The same rules apply if you are researching a group of primary care workers. How many are there? Over what geographical area? If your subjects are new referrals to a clinic, look at past referral data to find out the weekly/monthly/annual number of new referrals.

# Approach

Your method of approach will probably depend on the way you select your subjects. To recruit young people with asthma you might inform them of the study at an asthma clinic, although it is important to be aware that this method would restrict your sample to those already receiving certain services. If you are interested in a particular age group, you may be able to take a random sample from a register of patients, in which case you would probably write to those selected, inviting them to take part. Piloting your method of approach is not a bad idea if you think you might have trouble persuading people to take part.

## Exercise 7

Potential participants are likely to have a very different view of a piece of research than that of a funding body. Make a list of three good reasons for people to take part in your study. Now think of possible reasons why people may refuse. Use this information to compose a letter inviting a potential participant to take part in your study.

## Data collection

This part of the process takes place at the interface between researcher and subject, and as such can make or break the project. Therefore piloting your data collection tools is essential. The tools you use should be appropriate for the subject matter and the study design. They may include self-completion questionnaires, interviews (structured, semi-structured or qualitative interviews), clinical measurements (such as blood pressure or urinalysis) or a pro forma to obtain data from medical records. The key is to be consistent, particularly once the pilot phase is over, so try and avoid carrying out interviews in different locations (for example, home and surgery) or treating self-completed questionnaire data and interview data as if they were collected in the same way. Sometimes you have to be flexible and in these circumstances it is important to record the reasons for deviating from the study protocol.

## Data entry

This stage of the process should be considered at the time the data collection tools are designed. There are various computer software packages which facilitate the transition from questionnaire to data set but they still require human effort to input the information. Coding of questions should be clear and unambiguous and any decision about the most appropriate code must be made before data entry takes place. Researchers not entering their own data should bear in mind that another person undertaking this task is unlikely to be as obsessive and passionate about the overall project, therefore failure to ensure that data entry is a smooth procedure is likely to result in a loss of accuracy.

## Data checking

So you have got your data on file and you can start analysis, right? Wrong! With the research process well underway, it is inevitable that errors will have crept in at some stage and the first thing you need to do is look for obvious errors. These will include looking for contradictory situations (for example, cases where marital status is given as 'single' and source of social support is 'spouse', or cases where date of death falls before date of last consultation) and checking for extreme values (for example, people with a diastolic blood pressure of less than 40 mmHg).

## Data analysis

Whole books are devoted to this subject so this chapter will only touch on the kind of activities that take place and hurdles encountered during this stage of the research process. The type of analysis carried out will be limited by the type of data collected. Abandon hope now of using qualitative techniques on self-completed questionnaires which only included closed questions, or using sophisticated statistical techniques on transcribed, loosely structured interviews. As a general rule of thumb, start simple and build up. Describe the sample in terms of demographic characteristics (number of men and women, distribution across age groups, etc.). You are probably going to need to report this anyway when it comes to writing up but it will also help you familiarise yourself with the data set. When you want to start looking at differences between groups (for example, is alcohol consumption higher in those living in rural rather than non-rural areas?) or identify predictors for certain events (for example, what factors are associated with falls among the elderly?), you may need the help of a statistician. A statistician will be able to tell you whether certain tests are appropriate for the data you are working with, whereas a statistical package will uncritically carry out whatever you ask of it. What a statistician will not provide is a clinical interpretation of the findings. This has to come from your understanding of the subject area and familiarity with the way the study was carried out.

*Exercise 8*

Think ahead to the sort of paper you hope to write once the research has been carried out. Obviously you will not have any results until the data is collected, entered onto a computer, as appropriate, and analysed. However you should be able to anticipate the type of results you would like to present. Make a list of the titles of three tables you want to include (for example, 'Response by age and sex'; 'Baseline characteristics for intervention and control groups'). Use published papers of studies with a similar design to give you some ideas. The purpose of this activity is to reinforce the centrality of your research question throughout the process and to alert you to the kind of data you are going to need to collect.

## Writing up

A good research paper or report will be a good read and carry some sort of message. If the research question was important in the first place then it should make no difference whether the message is positive or negative (for example, a new and exciting intervention may have been found to be no more effective than the existing treatment or management). Ideally, a paper should be able to satisfy both the busy clinician who is looking to see how the study's findings might affect his or her practice, and the academic who is likely to subject the methods section to closer scrutiny. One of the reasons why researchers find writing up the most difficult part of the research process is because they are trying to write for an audience who has not lived and breathed the entire project from beginning to end. A fine line needs to be negotiated between including all the relevant parts of the conduct and findings of the study, without becoming bogged down in superfluous detail or being highly selective and misleading.

If you have been carrying out the activities in this section then you have already started to write up your research by giving yourself a framework for the background, methods and results section. Just because writing up is at the end of the research process does not mean that you should only start writing once every other part of the process is complete. Writing should be ongoing throughout the project. That way it becomes a less daunting task. For further help with the task of writing up, see Chapter 5 'Presenting and disseminating research'.

# Who funds research?

## Types of funding

Research funding varies in terms of source, size, purpose and the sort of strings that are attached to it. At this stage it is worth considering funding from two dimensions. Firstly, research can be purchaser (i.e. funding body) or provider (i.e. researcher) determined. Secondly, the investment of funds may be in the project itself or in the person carrying out the work. By taking these two dimensions together, it is possible to construct four broad categories of ways to secure funding for doing research (Figure 1.1).

Opportunistic funding is the type of research funding that those new to research are likely to be most familiar with. Research ideas are built up into a proposal, a suitable funding body is identified and the funding body responds to the grant application. It is essentially provider determined and project centred.

Commissioned research is also project centred but the need is identified by the purchaser rather than the provider. The NHS Research and Development Programme was introduced in 1991 to allow the NHS Executive to commission R&D directly on behalf of the NHS. Research needs are identified on the basis of national priorities such as *The Health of the Nation* targets. Calls for proposals appear periodically in the national press and professional journals.

Research fellowships, scholarships and training awards are funds invested in the researcher (person centred) rather than the project. Grant-making bodies will respond to a proposal for established or potential researchers to fund a piece of research to be carried out by the applicant, or for the applicant to undertake formal training in research skills. The nature of the fellowship or training is likely to be put together by the applicant in the form of a proposal and as such is provider determined.

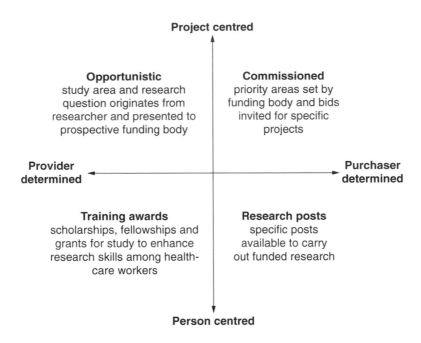

**Figure 1.1**  Getting research funded

The fourth way to get paid to do research is to get yourself a research job. Once commissioned or opportunistic funding is obtained, grant-holders are in the position to advertise for staff to carry out the research. Research posts are therefore determined by the grant-holder (now in the role of purchaser) as funds have been awarded for a specific piece of work.

## Main funding organisations

### Within the NHS

The NHS R&D Programme has both a central programme (discussed above) and eight regional programmes. This can be illustrated with reference to the Trent region where there are three sources of regional R&D funding:

- The Trent Research Scheme responds to ideas from researchers and is an example of opportunistic funding. Applications are invited twice a year.
- The Health Services Research (HSR) Training Awards Scheme aims to develop the capability and capacity of NHS professionals to undertake, understand and apply HSR in practice.
- Commissioned programmes cover work in areas which have been identified nationally and/or locally as priorities.

If you work for an NHS trust you should contact the local R&D officer. Many trusts now run annual research fellowship schemes, not least through Culyer funding which underpins much of the trust-based research initiatives in collaboration with local universities.

## Research councils

Two major research councils which fund primary care research are the Medical Research Council (MRC) and the Economic and Social Research Council (ESRC).

The Medical Research Council has an annual budget of around £300 million for funding medical and related biological research. The main funding schemes are project grants, programme grants, studentships and fellowships.

The Economic and Social Research Council funds research in all areas relating to the understanding of social and economic change. Award types vary and include project grants, research centres, research programmes and fellowships.

## Charities

Medical research charities and more general charities provide project grants, studentships and travel grants. Grants tend to be awarded on their relevance to the charity's particular area of interest. The following publications should be consulted. They can be found in the reference section of most university libraries.

- *Directory of Grant-making Trusts 1997–98* (1997). Charities Aid Foundation, Tonbridge.
- *A Guide to the Major Trusts* (1995). Directory of Social Change, London.
- *The Grants Register 1995–1997* (1994). Macmillan, London.
- *The Association of Medical Research Charities Handbook 1995–1996* (1995). AMRC, London.

## Professional bodies

Depending on your professional background, it is worth contacting your professional body for details of funding schemes currently available. Here are a few examples:

- The Scientific Foundation Board is the funding arm of the Royal College of General Practitioners, and supports research projects relevant to general practice. Awards are not exclusive to college members or general practitioners although priority may be given to these groups. First-time researchers are actively encouraged.
- The British Medical Association has a number of research awards and fellowships for scientists and medical practitioners available for application each year.
- The College of Occupational Therapists makes a number of small awards each year for education, research and continuing professional development.
- The Physiotherapy Research Foundation has a research project grant scheme, the primary aim of which is to support the development of research in physiotherapy and

to pump-prime projects. Grants of up to £10 000 are awarded although most awards are between £500 and £5000.

- The Bounty Health Visitor professional development awards are open to any practising member of the Health Visitors' Association and cover the costs of items such as course fees and conferences fees.

The English National Board for Nursing, Midwifery and Health Visiting does not respond to provider-determined applications but does commission research. It is shortly to produce a document on funding opportunities for nurses, midwives and health visitors.

# Putting together a grant application

With your research ideas sketched out in the activities in the first section, you should now be able to put a first draft of a research proposal together. Most funding bodies will have their own application forms and guide for applicants. This should be read carefully and if you are unsure about any part of the application form or guidelines then it is best to contact the funding body direct. The front sheet will usually be a summary sheet asking for the names of the applicant(s), the total funds sought, proposed starting date and duration of project and a short space for the project title and summary.

The next section will ask you for details of the proposed investigation and most funding bodies will break this down under certain headings. A typical layout is given below and the kind of information you should be providing is described. Not all of the *do's* and *don'ts* will apply to your own research but as you are going through the different sections of the application form, start to sort your own notes under the same headings.

## Aims of the project

This should be a clear and succinct statement of the research question(s).

*DO* make it obvious that the study is setting out to discover something.
*DO* refer back to the aims constantly in the other sections of the grant application.
*DON'T* state more than three aims. They should be memorable without the referee having to keep referring back to see what the applicant's aims were.

## Background to the project

This is a mini literature review. It is your chance to demonstrate the need for your study in terms of the importance of the issue and lack of evidence elsewhere.

*DO* keep it brief and refer to key literature.
*DO* demonstrate the timeliness of the proposed study.

*DON'T* attempt to show how widely read you are. The important thing is to keep the review focused.

*DON'T* rubbish other work in the field (it is impolite and may have been carried out by researchers who will be sent your application to review!).

## Study design

This may be, for example, an RCT, cross-sectional survey, case–control or qualitative study. If there is more than one phase to the study (for example, a cross-sectional survey followed by an RCT involving a subsection of the survey sample), now is the time to identify these as Phase 1 and Phase 2 and consistently refer to them as such during the remainder of the application.

*DO* describe the design in broad terms.

*DON'T* go into too much detail on the actual methods to be employed. This comes later.

## Methods

This part of the application will probably be the longest section. If the form does not do it for you, it may be useful to break it down into a series of subheadings yourself.

### Study population

You need to be very explicit about who will be eligible for the study and who will not be. Try and think of all potential recruits to the study and how your eligibility criteria should be drawn. The study setting should be stated clearly (for example, hospital admissions, out-patients, general practice, community dwelling, nursing home residents) and the appropriateness for using such a population should be justified.

*DO* state what type of sample you are taking (random, stratified random or non-random) and the sampling fraction(s) you intend to use.

*DON'T* be coy about the fact that you are not taking a random sample if it is inappropriate, impossible or unethical. If your sample is not random, there should be good reasons for this and you should state them confidently.

### Sample size calculation

You should state how many people you estimate to be included in the study and on what information you have based your estimate. This may be from audit information, previous research or pilot studies. Not using available information will give the impression that you are not as familiar as you should be with the literature and/or the service that you intend to study.

*DO* add in a factor for non-response and subjects dropping out of the study before the end-point.
*DON'T* give a whole series of longhand calculations – the application is likely to go to a statistical referee who will check this.

## Approach and consent

These are not just issues of concern to the local ethics committee, grant application referees will also want to know that this has been thought through in advance. Mode of approach (telephone, clinic staff, letter) and how informed consent will be obtained should be stated.

*DO* justify unorthodox modes of approach and demonstrate that you have considered their acceptability to subjects.
*DON'T* underestimate the burden on staff not directly involved in the study. If you are relying on them to approach potential subjects, then you need to make this as easy as possible for them.

## For RCTs

There are certain details that will need to be explained if the proposed study is an RCT. The unit of randomisation (individual, household, clinic), the point of randomisation (directly following recruitment, following interview, etc.) and the method of randomisation (sealed envelopes, phoning back to a central point) are all decisions to be made prior to commencement of the study. The intervention(s) should be described and it should be made clear how the arms of the trial differ from each other.

*DO* consider using a pathway diagram to demonstrate how recruits will pass through the study. (This may also apply to other complex study designs.)
*DON'T* forget to mention who will be 'blind' in the trial (subject, assessor, clinician).

## Assessment and instruments

About the assessment generally, the referees are going to need to know where it will take place (in the subject's home, in hospital, etc.), by whom or what (a lay interviewer, clinical interviewer, postal questionnaire, etc.), how long the assessment is likely to take and whether any follow-up assessments are planned. The instruments used during the assessment will need to be stated and justified in terms of their suitability for the task. If the instruments have been validated in a similar population then you should cite this work. Be very specific about your main outcome measure(s), and again, demonstrate its suitability to fulfil the aim(s) of the study.

*DO* give reasons for using non-standard instruments.
*DON'T* list instruments without stating what you intend to measure with them.
*DON'T* use abbreviations for measures without defining them.

*Statistical analysis*

For certain types of study (for example, RCTs with two arms and one binary outcome measure), the analysis may be self-explanatory but for other study designs you may wish to give a brief statement of the techniques you intend to use.

*DO* remember that the use of statistical analysis is not the main aim of health services research but to serve the aims of the study.
*DON'T* be overtechnical. You can cite references to support the use of non-standard techniques.

# Time-scale

Think this through carefully. The parts of the research process that take time are usually those that are outside of the direct control of the researcher, including gaining permission to carry out research in clinical settings, recruiting research staff and arranging meetings with project advisors from different organisations. Allow sufficient time at the beginning of the study period for preparing assessment instruments and recruiting subjects, and allow time at the end for writing up.

*DO* consider using a diagram with project milestones clearly marked.
*DO* be realistic about what you (and others) can achieve.
*DON'T* organise the time-scale in such a way that recruitment or posting questionnaires will occur around times of the year when many people are away (for example, just before Christmas and during summer holidays).

# Resources and costing

This part will be picked over with a fine-tooth comb by the grant-making body and referees. Careful and accurate costing of the component parts of the project will give the impression that the applicant has a clear idea as to the resource needs of the proposed study. Depending on the size of the project you should use subheadings where appropriate for staff, equipment and other running costs. The research office of community trusts, or the general practice manager, should be able to assist with this.

*DO* consult the grant-making body's guide for this as they may state specifically the kind of costs they are willing and unwilling to fund.
*DON'T* forget travel costs, photocopying, telephone costs, library charges and consultancy fees.

## Likely benefits of proposed research

This is extremely important. A beautifully designed study with no potential practical (either clinical or managerial) or theoretical gain is clearly not worth funding. State how the findings will affect decision making in delivering health services. Where possible, give an estimate of the numbers of service users or service providers who will be potentially affected by the health issue you are investigating.

*DO* make the connection between your study and current policy initiatives.
*DO* think about potential cost savings in terms of disease burden, economic and hidden costs (for example, burden on carers).
*DON'T* be shy at this point – you may be acting locally, but start to think nationally, if not globally!

## The ability of the applicant(s) to carry out the study

This part can be off-putting for first-time researchers as the implication is that the applicants should have a proven track record. This may be true for large projects to be carried out over a number of years by a team of dedicated researchers. However, for smaller projects the applicant should be able to demonstrate that the field of study is an area of their particular interest. This might be shown through the applicant's curriculum vitae in terms of professional rather than academic experience.

*DO* think about what is unique to your position for carrying out the proposed study.
*DO* contact experts in the field and ask if they would consider formal collaboration or acting as advisors to the study.
*DON'T* undersell your clinical experience and useful contacts.

## Dissemination

The whole point of carrying out research into healthcare is to improve the way services are delivered. Therefore findings from the research have to be communicated to those who need to know. The most obvious way this is done is through publication in a suitable journal, but speaking at relevant conferences and feeding back findings to local service providers and subjects who helped with the project should also be considered.

*DO* try and be imaginative at this stage. Publication in academic journals alone is probably not enough.
*DON'T* lose sight of local implications. You might want to organise a special workshop for these groups.

*Exercise 9*

The purpose of the exercise is to get you to think about how a referee, asked to review your grant application, might approach this task. What you should be getting a feel for is that good grant applications share certain characteristics. Try to judge your own application by using the following criteria:

- Is there a clear, researchable question?
- Does the project appear well thought through?
- Is it an important area?
- Is the project timely?
- Are the findings likely to be generalisable?
- What is the potential value to the field of knowledge?
- What is the potential practical value?
- How appropriate is the overall study design?
- How suitable are the methods/measures to be used?

It is often hard to assess your own work so ask a colleague for their frank opinion of your proposal. Have you got your message across?

# Summary

## Give yourself time

The process of obtaining research funds takes longer than you think. Most grant-making bodies will have deadlines for applications at certain times each year. Do not under-estimate how long it will take to put your application together. Many of the hold-ups (for example, waiting to meet people who will be able to grant you access to potential subjects) will be out of your control. You should also get others to read it through to check the main messages are getting across to the reader.

## Know what is going on

You need to be aware of changes in health policy, nationally and locally. Read the news section of your professional journals and pay attention to health issues reported on national and local media. A research study does not exist in a vacuum but in the ever-changing world of health service provision. When you write your application you need to show how your study fits in to the bigger picture.

## Dealing with rejection

Putting together a decent application for funding involves a lot of hard work and if it is unsuccessful then this can be a major blow to the applicant. Try not to despair, or harbour resentment against the referees whose comments should have been returned with the application.

If the grant-making body is prepared to consider a resubmitted proposal (amended along the lines of the referees' comments) then you have to consider whether this can be done. Generally, persistence pays off. Clearly, the funding body is interested and if there are good reasons not to change certain aspects of the proposed study then justify this in the resubmission. It may be that the referees have misunderstood the proposed study, in which case you need to improve the clarity of the application.

If the negative response was more final, then you might consider an alternative funding body. It is still worth taking on board the referees' comments. Referees are likely to be experts in the field and their insight should be valued. Another option is to consider applying for funds for a pilot study. If a smaller pilot study rather than the definitive piece of research is proposed, it will inevitably be seen as a less risky investment of funds by the grant-making body.

# Answers to exercises

Since the exercises for this chapter are to a large extent based on self-selected examples, it is not feasible to provide specific answers to the exercises. You should, however, draw on the guidelines provided in the text when approaching them.

# References

Department of Health (1997) *Research and Development: Towards an Evidence-based Health Service.* The Stationery Office, London.

Mead D (1997) Research grant myths quashed. *Nursing Times.* **93**: 19, 53.

Singh N, Clements K and Fiatarone M (1997) A randomized controlled trial of progressive resistance training in depressed elders. *Journal of Gerontology.* **52A**: M27–M35.

# Further reading and resources

## General texts

In addition to the references cited in this chapter, the following general texts have sections on the research process and many include information on obtaining funding.

Brink P J and Wood M J (1994) *Basic Steps in Planning Nursing Research: From Question to Proposal.* Jones and Bartlett, Boston.

Carter Y and Thomas C (1997) *Research Methods in Primary Care.* Radcliffe Medical Press, Oxford.

Crombie I K and Davies H T O (1996) Research in Health Care: Design, Conduct and Interpretation of Health Services Research. Wiley, Chichester.

Hicks C (1995) *Research for Physiotherapists: Project Design and Analysis.* Churchill Livingston, Edinburgh.

## Reports and papers

The following publications will give a background to the development of R&D in the NHS.

Culyer A (1994) *Supporting Research and Development in the NHS.* HMSO, London.

Department of Health (1993) *Research for Health.* DoH, London.

Department of Health (1996) *Research and Development: Towards an Evidence-based Health Service Information Pack.* DoH, London.

The National Association of Health Authorities and Trusts (NAHAT) has produced a series of discussion papers on health service issues, including the role of research in primary care. They can be contacted at the following address:

NAHAT
Birmingham Research Park
Vincent Drive
Birmingham B15 2SQ
Tel: 0121 471 4444

## Addresses of other organisations mentioned in the text

Board of Science and Education
British Medical Association
Tavistock Square
London WC1H 9JP
Tel: 0171 383 6351

College of Occupational Therapists
6–8 Marshalsea Road
London SE1 1HL
Tel: 0171 357 6480

Community Practitioners and Health Visitors' Association
50 Southwark Street
London SE1 1UN
Tel: 0171 717 4000

Economic and Social Research Council
Polaris House
North Star Avenue
Swindon SN2 1UJ
Tel: 01793 413000

English National Board for Nursing, Midwifery and Health Visiting
Victory House
170 Tottenham Court Road
London W1P 0HA
Tel: 0171 388 3131

Medical Research Council
20 Park Crescent
London W1N 4AL
Tel: 0171 636 5422

NHS R&D Programme
NHS Executive
Quarry House
Quarry Hill
Leeds LS2 7UE
Tel: 0113 254 5000

Physiotherapy Research Foundation
Chartered Society of Physiotherapy
14 Bedford Row
London WC1R 4ED
Tel: 0171 306 6666

Research & Development Group
NHS Executive, Trent
Fulwood House
Old Fulwood Road
Sheffield S10 3TH
Tel: 0114 282 0332

Scientific Foundation Board
Royal College of General Practitioners
14 Princes Gate
Hyde Park
London SW7 1PU
Tel: 0171 581 3232

## Acknowledgements

The author wishes to thank Andrew Booth at the School of Health and Related Research, University of Sheffield and the Trent Institute for Health Services Research for providing information on research funding; Beverly Hancock from Trent Focus for providing initial guidance on the content of the chapter; and Julie McGarry for reading through early drafts.

# CHAPTER TWO

# Carrying out a literature review

*Michael Hewitt*

## Introduction

The aim of this chapter is to provide an introduction to 'reviewing the literature'. After working through the chapter you will be able to:

- appreciate the role of the literature review in the research process
- conduct a literature search
- develop skills to critically review research literature
- write a literature review.

This chapter defines some key terminology and presents an overview of the process of the literature review.

## What is meant by the 'literature'?

In professional and academic disciplines the term 'literature' is used to describe all the published work on a particular subject. Within this definition, no judgement is made regarding the quality of any single piece of work.

The main corpus of the literature lies within academic and professional journals. It has been estimated that about 20 000 journals published each year carry articles that are relevant to the disciplines of the medical and health sciences.

## What is a literature review?

A literature review is a self-contained piece of written work that gives a concise summary of previous findings in an area of the research literature. It reflects an author's knowledge and interpretation of the area of interest. It has a reference section that lists the individual pieces of work referred to in the review. Like all pieces of written research output it should include a description of the methods used to create the work.

Literature reviews vary considerably in their depth and breadth, as well as style of presentation, depending on the purpose intended by the author. This may range from a superficial search of the literature to give a researcher an insight to an area of potential research through to a scientifically rigorous 'systematic review'.

Researchers committed to writing a review, however, should be encouraged to go beyond superficial searches and simply listing research works or they will inevitably get a biased or incomplete view of the research area under investigation. Instead, they should develop skills that will enable them to systematically search for literature and critically review the research uncovered by the search. This chapter aims to help primary healthcare professionals achieve these skills.

## Why do a literature review?

In general, the research process follows a number of distinct stages. Before any actual research can take place there are a number of planning stages to consider. Figure 2.1 shows a schematic representation of possible planning stages and their relationship to the full research process.

Central to the planning stages is the literature review. A preliminary review of the literature will help in further identifying and clarifying your research problem. A little further down the line it may provide the theoretical input to your research idea and help in the formulation of the research question. More specifically, a literature review will:

*   provide an up-to-date picture of the research area of interest and show which areas have been investigated and the results obtained
*   identify methods of investigation that could be used in further research
*   give indications of problems that might be encountered and possible solutions
*   reveal common findings among studies
*   reveal inconsistencies between studies
*   identify factors not previously considered
*   provide suggestions for further research.

## How is a literature review done?

The process of carrying out a literature review can be described by three actions. These are searching, reviewing and writing. All three actions are outlined below and covered in later sections in more detail.

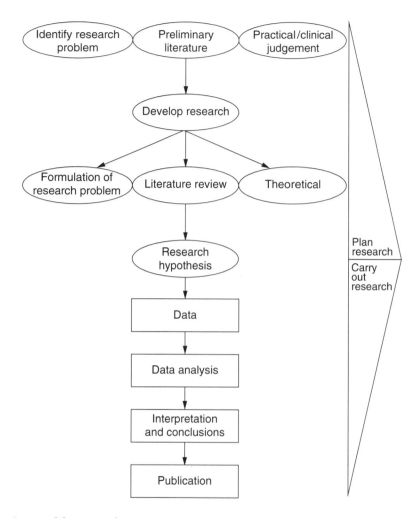

**Figure 2.1**    Stages of the research process

Searching requires a trip to a medical library and, in the early stages, the assistance of a librarian is particularly helpful. It involves scanning a range of information resources and careful recording of different searches and outputs. The literature yield from searching is likely to be of variable relevance and quality. The next stage in the process is, therefore, to critically assess each work along relevance and quality dimensions. Finally, it is important to document the whole process. This includes how the search was performed and how the literature was assessed in terms of the aforementioned dimensions. The body of the report summarises the main findings presented in the literature and highlights areas of agreements, inconsistencies or areas where more research is needed.

## Published literature reviews

Examples of published literature reviews include Fletcher *et al.* (1997) on compression treatment for venous leg ulcers, Hallam (1994) on out-of-hours primary medical care, Liu *et al.* (1990) on combined insulin–glibenclamide therapy for NIDDM patients, Roberts *et al.* (1996) on the role of health visiting in the prevention of childhood injury, Weinberg (1990) on asthma and Wood (1991) on antenatal care in primary care settings.

## Summary

This section has presented an overview of reviewing the literature. The following sections look in more detail at the process. The next section examines the publication of primary healthcare research. It describes in more detail what is meant by the literature and how a piece of research becomes a part of this body of knowledge. This is followed by two sections describing the methods that have been devised for selecting out particular subsets of the literature. The next section describes a step-by-step approach to planning and conducting a literature search. The final section provides an overview of how to process the results of your literature search and turn them into a review. To assist the learning process, practical exercises are provided at key stages of the chapter. These take you through the essential steps of conducting your own review.

# The publication of primary healthcare research

The main source of literature used for a review is articles published in journals. Other sources of literature, however, need to be considered and these include books, reports, conference proceedings, theses and dissertations. This section provides an overview of how and where research findings are published.

## Journals

The final step of the research process (Figure 2.1) requires that research findings be published. This is necessary for two main reasons. First, so that the findings are open to critical examination by others, and second, that they are accessible to all who might benefit from them. The traditional vehicle for publishing research findings is journals.

Journals are magazine-sized publications containing articles. They are published in issues at regular intervals, usually weekly, monthly or quarterly. Because of the regularity of publication they are also known as periodicals or serials. This regularity means that each new issue contains articles that describe the latest research findings; this is a distinct advantage over other publication media such as books which take longer to produce and update.

The publication of an article in a journal involves a number of steps:

(1)   *writing the article* – this requires the author or authors to present their research findings in a broadly scientific style. The layout of the article may also need to conform to a particular style laid down by the editorial board of the journal; this may require the authors to include a summary (or abstract) of their work, or to keep within a specified word limit, for example

(2)   *submission of the article to a journal* – usually via the journal's editor

(3)   *refereeing* – some journals require that articles are critically reviewed by experts in the field prior to publication. This process is also known as 'peer review'. Referees may suggest amendments to the original text before publication can proceed, or may reject the article outright if they argue the work is fatally flawed in some way

(4)   *changes to the original text* – if indicated by the referees

(5)   *publication* – if, or when, the editor accepts the article.

There are basically two main types of journal:

*   research journals
*   professional journals.

Research journals publish peer-reviewed articles. A few examples of the many thousands of research journals available include the *British Medical Journal*, the *Lancet* and the *British Journal of General Practice*. In contrast, professional journals publish articles on professional issues, service developments, the use of research findings in practice and some short research articles. They are primarily written for practising healthcare professionals rather than researchers. Examples include the *Health Visitor Journal*, the *Journal of District Nursing* and *Practice Nurse*.

## Reports

Research reports appear in many different shapes and sizes. In general, however, they will give a more detailed account of a piece of research than that found in a journal article. Reports of original research may arise from many different sources, including health authorities, professional organisations and pharmaceutical companies. The publicity and distribution of some reports may be very limited, making it difficult to know of them or obtain copies.

## Theses and dissertations

Theses and dissertations are very detailed and comprehensive accounts of research work. They are usually submitted for a higher degree at a university. Like reports, their publicity and distribution may be very limited.

# Conference proceedings

Conference proceedings comprise brief summaries of research work presented at conferences. Researchers sometimes use conferences to present preliminary findings of their work. A more detailed and complete account of the work may appear at a later date in a journal article, report or thesis.

# Books

Textbooks generally provide comprehensive overviews of a particular subject. In doing so they may refer to, sometimes extensively, the research literature found in journal articles, reports, conference proceedings or theses. They are not usually used to present new research findings. There are, however, a few exceptions to this and some very important and influential research findings have been published in book format. These are sometimes known as research monographs.

# Summary

Primary healthcare research is published in a variety of formats, including journal articles, books, reports, conference proceedings, theses and dissertations. The first stage of the literature review is to locate all the research findings on a particular subject from the literature, regardless of the publication format. The next section shows how this can be achieved.

## *Exercise 1*

1. The publication process

Locate one or two journals that present articles written by healthcare professionals or researchers. Look for information on the publication of articles within each journal (this may be presented as instructions for authors or may be found with the general information about the journal or editors located on the front inside cover). Use the information to answer the following questions:

* Is there a limit to the number of words each article must not exceed?
* Are the articles peer-reviewed?
* Should each article include an abstract?
* How should references be presented?
* Can the article be submitted on a floppy disc?

2. Relevant literature

List any journals you know of that are likely to contain articles relevant to your profession. Add to the list any relevant reports, theses, conference proceedings and books.

# Bibliographic tools to locate published research

A key stage in the literature review is to search out all the research literature on a particular subject. This may at first seem an impossible task given the huge volume of research literature published worldwide. This problem, however, has long been recognised and considerable effort has been made to simplify and speed up the process. The results of this effort are known as 'bibliographic tools'. This section describes the main bibliographic tools used to locate published research and how to use them.

## Bibliographic tools: journals

The main bibliographic tools for locating journal articles are indexing journals and abstracting journals.

### Indexing journals

Indexing journals tell you what has been published and where. They are published like journals but contain lists of references to journal articles, not articles themselves. A reference provides basic information about a published work such as who wrote it, the title, which journal it was published in and when. An example of a reference is:

Brown M and Olshansky E (1997) From limbo to legitimacy: a theoretical model of the transition to the primary care nurse practitioner role. *Nursing Research.* **46**(1): 46–51.

The references in an index are listed under different subject headings. Some indexes have a large number of subject headings that represent the majority of key terms or concepts that appear in the medical and health sciences literature. A few of the many key terms relevant to primary healthcare could include: general practice, practice nurse, primary healthcare, community nursing.

In producing an index a publishing company has scanned a large number of journals, noting the reference of each article found. Each article is tagged with a number of permitted key terms that best describe the contents. The reference to each article is then published in the index under each major key term (subject heading) carried by it. As an example, the reference above could be best described by the following key terms: practice nurse, primary healthcare, nursing: theory. The reference would be listed under those headings in the published index.

There are several indexes that cover journals relevant to primary healthcare research. These include *Index Medicus*, the *Cumulative Index to Nursing and Allied Health Literature*, the *Nursing and Midwifery Index*, the *Nursing Bibliography* and the *International Nursing Index*. A brief outline of each is presented below.

*Index Medicus. Index Medicus* is one of the largest indexing journals. It covers a wide range of the international biomedical and medicine-related literature. Information is currently indexed from about 3700 journals. It lists references under an extensive system of subject headings known as MeSH (medical subject headings). It is published monthly with annual cumulative editions.

*Cumulative Index to Nursing and Allied Health Literature* (CINAHL). CINAHL covers about 300 journals in the nursing and related health fields. It is published bimonthly with annual cumulative editions.

*Nursing and Midwifery Index* (NMI). NMI covers about 150 journals in nursing and midwifery. It is published monthly with annual cumulative editions. In 1997 the index was retitled the *British Nursing Index* (BNI).

*Nursing Bibliography.* This is a monthly index published by the Royal College of Nursing (RCN). It covers the journals held in the RCN library.

*International Nursing Index* (INI). INI covers about 600 journals on nursing, midwifery and health visiting. It is published quarterly with annual cumulative editions.

## Abstracting journals

Abstracting journals are similar to indexing journals in that they tell you what has been published and where. They differ, however, in the information they publish. Whereas indexing journals publish references to articles they have found, abstracting indexes publish each reference with an accompanying abstract. The abstract summarises the full written work.

Research journals commonly require authors to submit abstracts with their full article. They are usually printed at the beginning of each article when published. An example of an entry in an abstracting journal is:

Neil H A W, Roe L, Godlee R J P, Moore J W, Clark G M G, Brown J, Thorogood M, Stratton I M, Lancaster T, Mant D, Fowler G H
Randomised trial of lipid-lowering dietary advice in general practice: The effects on serum lipids, lipoproteins, and antioxidants.
*British Medical Journal*, 1995, Vol. 310, No.6979, pp. 569–573.
Objective – To determine the relative efficacy in general practice of dietary advice given by a dietitian, a practice nurse, or a diet leaflet alone in reducing total and low-density lipoprotein cholesterol concentration.
Design – Randomised six-month parallel trial.
Setting – A general practice in Oxfordshire.
Subjects – 2004 subjects aged 35–64 years were screened for hypercholesterolaemia; 163 men and 146 women with a repeat total cholesterol concentration of 6.0–8.5 mmol/l entered the trial.

Interventions – Individual advice provided by a dietitian using a diet history, a practice nurse using a structured food frequency questionnaire, or a detailed diet leaflet sent by post. All three groups were advised to limit the energy provided by fat to 30% or less and to increase carbohydrate and dietary fibre.

Main outcome measures – Concentrations of total cholesterol and low-density and high-density lipoprotein cholesterol after six months; antioxidant concentration and body mass index.

Results – No significant differences were found at the end of the trial between groups in mean concentrations of lipids, lipoproteins, and antioxidants or body mass index. After data were pooled from the three groups, the mean total cholesterol concentration fell by 1.9% (0.13 mmol/l, 95% confidence interval 0.06 to 0.22, $p < 0.001$) to 7.00 mmol/l, and low-density lipoprotein cholesterol also fell. The total carotenoid concentration increased by 53 mmol/l (95% confidence interval 3.0 to 103, $p = 0.039$).

Conclusions – Dietary advice is equally effective when given by a dietitian, a practice nurse, or a diet leaflet alone but results in only a small reduction in total and low-density lipoprotein cholesterol. To obtain a better response more intensive intervention than is normally available in primary care is probably necessary.

An abstract of an article is useful additional information to have. It may help when assessing the relevance of the research work to your particular area of interest without the need for the full article. We shall return to this issue later in the final section 'Examining the results and writing a review', p. 47.

The main abstracting journal for medical sciences is known as *Excerpta Medica*. It covers about 4700 journals (including some book reviews and conference proceedings) from the biomedical literature. It has a strong coverage of European research and the pharmaceutical literature. *Excerpta Medica* is published as a series of 51 sections on different medical topics; each is published monthly with annual cumulative editions.

# Bibliographic tools: other sources of literature

Although the majority of literature for a review will be journal based, you may need to trace material in other formats such as books. If this is the case then a different set of bibliographic tools must be used. These include bibliographies and library catalogues.

## *Bibliographies*

Bibliographies do for books and other formats of literature what indexes do for journals. The major bibliography for books currently in print is called *Whitaker's Books in Print*. Books are arranged in alphabetical order separately for authors and titles as well as a subject index. One major limitation is that not all publishers are represented. Another significant bibliography is the *British National Bibliography*, which is based on the stock of the British Library.

There are a small number of specialist bibliographies. The most notable one is the *Steinberg Collection of Nursing Research*, which is published by the Royal College of Nursing (RCN). It provides details of all theses held in the RCN library in London.

### Library catalogues

Library catalogues provide guidance to the literature available within a particular library. As well as books and conference proceedings they will list locally produced reports, dissertations and theses that are held in stock.

## Summary

Bibliographic tools have been developed to help locate research literature. There are a number of different indexing and abstracting journals (simply referred to as 'indexes') to help locate articles in journals. Other sources of literature can be located using bibliographies and library catalogues. The next section describes how to use the various bibliographic tools.

# How to use bibliographic tools

Most of the bibliographic tools described in the last section are available in two formats: paper and electronic. Searching the paper versions can take many hours of work, involving manually scanning the different indexing or abstracting journals. The electronic (or computerised) versions are relatively new but have already had a significant impact on the search process; what can take several hours of manual searching can be achieved in minutes with a computer.

There are two ways of searching the literature using a computer. The first is via 'CD-ROM' and the second is 'on-line'. With CD-ROM (compact disc read-only memory) the references to the literature are stored in digital form on compact discs, just like the ones used now for music recordings. The on-line method uses networks of electronically connected computers. A large remote computer is used to store the references and access to them is made via a local library computer. Most medical libraries will offer at least one of these services, with the assistance of a librarian if required.

The remainder of this section shows examples of manual and computerised searches. Manual searching is sometimes still required, as not every indexing or abstracting journal is available via CD-ROM or on-line.

# Manual search

Subject: Postnatal depression
Index: Vol. 6, No. 9, 1996 of the *Nursing and Midwifery Index* (NMI) will be searched.

1.  Check that postnatal depression is a subject heading used by NMI. The list of subject headings is located at the back of the issue.
2.  Find the heading in the main part of the index.
3.  Note the references:

     Barclay L and Lloyd B
     The misery of motherhood: alternative approaches to maternal distress. (17 refs.)
     *Midwifery*, 1996, Vol. 12, No. 3, pp. 136–139.

     Beck C
     A meta-analysis of the relationship between postpartum depression and infant temperament. (52 refs.)
     *Nursing Research*, 1996, Vol. 45, No. 4, pp. 225–230.

     Three more references are listed.

# CD-ROM search

This example shows a search of the MEDLINE CD-ROM. MEDLINE is the computerised version of *Index Medicus*, which is described in the previous section. The computerised version differs slightly from the original paper version in that it carries abstracts for most references.
Subject: The management of asthma in general practice
CD-ROM: MEDLINE 1987–1992. OVID Search Software Version 3.
The following keywords were entered in turn:

*   asthma
*   general practice.

The following is displayed on the screen:

```
Database: MEDLINE <1987 to 1992>

Set    Search                                                Results
-------------------------------------------------------------------
001    asthma/                                                10710
002    family practice/                                        6098
003    1 and 2                                                   69
```

For each keyword entered the computer generates a result which indicates the number of articles found. Notice that although the second keyword entered was 'general practice' the computer records it as 'family practice'. The change occurred as the search software mapped 'general practice' on to the preferred subject heading, i.e. family practice (*Index Medicus* is produced in the USA hence it uses American terminology and spellings). The final line requests that the first two keywords are combined in one search; that is, find only those articles that appear under both subject headings (69 in this case).

Each search set can be viewed and shows the reference to each article found together with the abstract. References and abstracts can be selected and printed out, or transferred electronically to other computer software such as databases and word-processing packages.

## On-line search

This example shows a search of the on-line service called EMBASE. This is the computerised version of *Excerpta Medica* which is described in the previous section.

Subject: The management of depression in general practice
Index: EMBASE on-line 1994–1996
A search using 'words in title' (selected via the on-screen menu) was carried out. The keywords entered were:

- depression
- general practice.

The two keywords were combined in a single search. This generated the following output:

```
3.  1994-1996              19        1+2
2.  1994-1996             885        (general practice)@TI
1.  1994-1996            3498        (depression)@TI
```

In this example, only references with the keywords in their title (indicated by the notation '@TI') were located. This is an alternative strategy for searching.

## General points on computer searching

Unlike manual searching, computer searching is an interactive process. The searcher types in a keyword on the keyboard, and the computer displays the result as the number of references retrieved. The references themselves can be seen when the user issues a 'display' or 'print' command. Usually the commands are available via an on-screen menu.

Computer searching offers a number of advantages over manual searching. First, it is very much quicker. Second, as demonstrated above, search terms can be combined in order to retrieve references listed under two or more subject headings. Third, you have the choice of using keywords that the index uses or you can use so-called 'free text' which can be any word or phrase. Free-text searches will retrieve references where the word or phrase appears anywhere in the title or abstract of an article.

## Summary

This section has briefly described how to use different bibliographic tools. In practice you will encounter many different indexes and computer systems; it is beyond the scope of this chapter to describe them all. The examples and exercises below are limited to those most commonly available. Learning how to use bibliographic tools is best achieved through practical experience in the library and becoming familiar with the systems available to you.

### Exercise 2

Most libraries will offer the assistance of a suitably experienced librarian when using bibliographic tools. Beginners are well advised to seek this assistance.

1.  Locating bibliographic tools
Medical libraries have a number of bibliographic tools available for general use. Visit your local library and find out which ones are held and in which format they are available (i.e. paper/electronic).

2.  Using bibliographic tools
Replicate the manual search on postnatal depression using the *Nursing and Midwifery Index* as described in this section.
Replicate the MEDLINE CD-ROM search on asthma in primary care as described in this section.

## Conducting a literature search

The objective of a literature search is to retrieve as much accurate information on a given subject as is possible from suitable sources. It is clear from this and the preceding sections that the novice reviewer is faced with a difficult task. The pool of available research literature is huge and only a tiny fraction of it, the particular subject of interest, needs to be located. Help is at hand of course in the form of bibliographic tools, but which ones should you use? And in which format – paper or electronic?

   This section presents some basic guidelines to follow when tackling a literature search. Like all types of investigation, an effective search requires careful planning. A badly organised search is likely to yield little relevant information and waste time.

## General points

The first point to note is that the planning stage is the same for both manual and computerised searching; only the mechanics of searching differ. Second, a search takes time to complete, even for the experienced reviewer. A reasonable, continuous period of time should be set aside for the task; an hour here or there is not sufficient. Third, it is important to be systematic and record each step of your search. With indexes or abstracting journals one useful approach is to start with the most recent and to work backwards. There are no hard and fast rules for the period of the search, except to say that it would be unwise to restrict it to recent years. Finally, decide on your subject of interest and stick to it during the search. When browsing through indexes many interesting-looking titles will appear – don't get sidetracked.

## Bibliographic tools

The choice of bibliographic tools may well depend on what your local library can offer. If possible then at least one computerised search (e.g. MEDLINE or EMBASE) should be performed. One general point to consider is the subject of interest and potential coverage by the different indexes. The main indexes cover much of the mainstream medical literature, but at the same time do not cover all of the journals in all disciplines. It is wise, therefore, to check the list of journals a particular index covers (this is published with each annual cumulative edition) before starting. If the most common journals in your field are missing then a search of that particular index may not be a good place to start. Furthermore, although MEDLINE and EMBASE cover over 3000 journals each, it has been estimated that there is only about a 30% overlap of journal coverage. If they are available then both should be searched.

## Keywords

To increase the chances of retrieving relevant information from a search, you need to create a description of the subject of interest. This takes the form of a set of words or phrases which are known as 'search terms' or 'keywords'. Each search term or keyword identifies a part of the subject and provides a focus for the search.

The process of creating keywords involves three stages:

(1)  identify the key concepts in your research area
(2)  analyse the concepts; extend their scope to find broader terms; define them with increasing precision to produce narrower terms; produce a list of synonyms; produce a list of related terms
(3)  map the list of keywords or terms to the subject headings of each index to be used in the search.

## Creating key terms: an example

The area of interest is health visiting and the prevention of accidents to children in the home. The key concepts are health visitor, accident prevention, children and home. To analyse the concepts it can help to create 'spider diagrams' as shown in Figure 2.2.

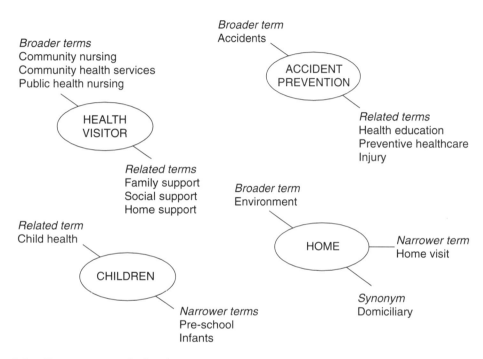

**Figure 2.2**   Key concepts and related terms

Start the diagram by writing down the key concepts on a blank piece of paper. Carry out a brainstorming activity and make a note of related, broader and narrower terms as well as synonyms for each one.

Having worked through these steps you will have a list of keywords that you can match to the subject headings used by the indexing journals. Examples of this are shown in Table 2.1. Keywords have been matched to subject headings from the *Nursing and Midwifery Index* (NMI).

The majority of indexes publish the subject headings they use. These are individual to each index. Some of your keywords will match exactly those used by a particular index (this includes a close match where the preferred subject heading will be suggested), some will match another, and others will not match at all.

**Table 2.1**  Keywords and matched NMI subject headings

| Keyword | NMI subject heading |
| --- | --- |
| Health visitor | Health visiting |
| Community nursing | Community nursing |
| Public health nursing | No match |
| Home support | Home care services |
| Family support | No match |
| Accident prevention | Accident prevention |
|  | Also Children: accidents |
| Children | Children |
| Infants | Infants |
| Pre-school | No match |

## Recording the results

The results of a search are references to articles. For manual searches you have no choice but to write out by hand every reference found. One useful way to do this is to use index cards. Enter each reference on a single card (Figure 2.3) and store in a box. This allows the references to be sorted in some meaningful way (e.g. alphabetically by author, or grouped into categories, etc.) at a later date.

Larson C P

Efficacy of prenatal and postpartum home visits on child health and development

*Pediatrics*, 1980, **66**,183–90.

**Figure 2.3**  An example index card

It is also important to record the progress of your search. This ensures a systematic approach. One way would be to compile a table which can be marked as required (Table 2.2).

Computerised searches will generate reference lists that can be transferred electronically on to a computer and loaded into a database or word processor. Alternatively,

**Table 2.2**   Framework for systematic recording of searches

| Index | Subject heading | Years searched | | | | | |
|---|---|---|---|---|---|---|---|
| | | 1996 | 1995 | 1994 | 1993 | 1992 | 1991 |
| *NMI* | Health visiting | ✓ | ✓ | | | | |
| | Accident prevention | ✓ | ✓ | | | | |
| | Accidents: children | ✓ | | | | | |
| *Index Medicus* | Community health nursing | | | | | | |
| | Accident prevention | | | | | | |
| | Child | | | | | | |

they can be printed out on paper. Computerised searches will also record your search details, as for example:

```
Database: Medline <1993 to April 1997>
Set    Search                                        Results
-------------------------------------------------------------------
001    community health nursing/                        2095
002    accident prevention/                              272
003    child/                                          97783
004    1 and 2 and 3                                        5
```

## Satisfactory searches

When conducting your search it is always a good idea to periodically examine the references and decide if the search is 'on target'. It is difficult, often impossible, to know how many references to expect on a particular subject. However, if you already know of some key references in the area and your search does not find these, you should suspect a problem.

There are a number of problems that can occur at each stage of the search process. For example, you may have:

- defined your subject too narrowly and ended up with no references
- defined your subject too broadly and ended up with thousands of references
- used inappropriate keywords
- chosen the wrong (or not the best) indexes for your search.

*Finding too little*: be especially careful if you find nothing. Often this is not the case. Proving that there is nothing is not easy. You should try several different approaches before coming to this conclusion. It is easier to begin a search with a broad strategy and narrow appropriately than to construct a narrow search and try to broaden it if you find nothing.

*Finding too much*: this is a common problem, particularly with computerised searching. Try limiting the search by selecting relevant subheadings for the search terms you are using.

If you decide your search is unsatisfactory then you need to revisit keyword and index selections and iterate through the process again.

# Summary

This section has provided an insight into conducting a literature search. To maximise the success of a search careful planning is required. Decisions need to be made, for instance concerning the bibliographic tools to be used and the time period to search. One important step is the construction of keywords to be used in searching; care here may save you time looking through irrelevant material later. Finally, it is important to record the searches you perform and the results.

The output from the literature search is a list of references to articles of the subject of your interest. If you have used some of the computerised bibliographic tools or have searched an abstracting journal, each reference is likely to include a summary (abstract) of the full article. The final section looks at how to analyse and review this literature.

*Exercise 3*

Plan and conduct a literature search.

1.  Decide on an area of interest for investigation. Try to think of a specific area/problem/feature/question of your work rather than a general area. For example, 'Are practice nurses effective in delivering healthcare?' is too general, whereas 'Do practice nurses give effective quit-smoking advice?' is more specific and a more appropriate starting place.
2.  Collect together any articles you may already have on the area of interest. Use the articles and your clinical experience in the area to make a list of key terms/phrases/concepts.
3.  Use the list of key terms and generate broader, narrower and related terms and synonyms (use spider diagrams as shown in Figure 2.2 if this helps).
4.  Make a list of the bibliographic tools that are available to you, for instance indexes such as MEDLINE and *NMI*.
5.  Match your list of key terms (from step c above) to the subject headings used by each index.
6.  Draw up a table of the index, subject headings and years to be searched (see Table 2.2 for an example).
7.  Conduct the search, be systematic and record all results carefully as described in the section.

# Examining the results and writing a review

Examining the results of a literature search can be performed at different levels of complexity. This may range from a superficial scan of the references to decide on relevance to a detailed analysis of the quality of each article. The aim of this section is to present an overview of these levels of analysis. The final part of the section outlines the structure of a literature review report.

## Relevance

The first level of analysis is to scan the list of references, remove duplicates and assess the relevance of the material your search produced. It is easier to assess relevance when using references from abstracting journals than indexing journals because a summary of the work is provided by the abstract.

However, assessing relevance on the strength of an abstract is not always possible and in some instances the full paper will be required. In addition, the quality of the material can only be assessed by looking at the original work. Collecting copies of original articles is therefore the next task and a visit to the nearest medical library is one place where a search can begin.

Medical libraries will publish a list of journals they subscribe to and a proportion of your references can be photocopied from stock. However, libraries have finite budgets and shelf space and will only hold a limited number of journals. It is not likely, therefore, that all of your references will be available from a single library. This problem is resolved by the inter-library loans (ILL) system whereby items from other libraries are lent or photocopied on request. Two important points must be made with regard to the ILL system. First, it takes time to process each request and provide the material; this delay can be as long as four weeks. Second, the ILL system is not free and a charge may be made for each item requested. Consult your local library staff for details.

## Quality

It is important to note that the contents of an article do not necessarily represent facts just because they are in print. An article may instead represent the views or opinions of an author which are not based on research evidence. Reading literature critically and assessing quality can be a complex and involved activity. It is a skill that needs to be learned, practised and developed. There are, however, a number of guidelines that can help you get started with this process.

*Peer review*

The first section described the steps involved in the publication process. One important stage in the process is peer review where each article is critically reviewed prior to publication. This acts as a filtering stage with the idea that only works of sufficient quality are published.

To some extent, therefore, you can judge an article by the journal in which it appears. Journals that use peer review will have an editorial committee and/or an editorial advisory board. They will outline their arrangements for peer review in each issue of the journal. This can usually be found on the inside front or back cover of the journal.

*Reading articles*

Before you consider a detailed analysis of each article it is worth previewing each one by scanning the abstract, introduction, headings and subheadings, tables and figures, discussion and conclusions and the reference list. This will provide you with an initial impression of the article – whether there are any obvious omissions, lack of detail, errors in presentation of figures. A reference list, for example, that includes articles from a range of journals and years, with books and other formats included, will indicate that a proper search of the literature has been made.

## Critical appraisal

Critical appraisal of research articles involves asking the question 'Am I persuaded by this study's results?'. Answering this question involves asking a series of other questions:

- Is the purpose of the study clear and well defined?
- How was the study done?
- Are the methods clearly described and appropriate?
- Are the results presented in a clear and understandable format?
- Does the interpretation of the results seem consistent with the results presented?
- Are there other explanations that could account for the results?

The above set of questions can be answered by a second set of more detailed questions. These take the form of check-lists which have been specifically developed to critically assess different types of research designs and articles (for instance, Crombie 1996).

## Writing a review

The structure of a review generally follows that of an original research article. It will have sections for methods, results, discussion and conclusions as well as an introduction.

The introduction should state the purpose of the review and give brief background information on the subject of the review. The methods section should describe in detail the methods used to compile the review. This will include details of which indexes were used, the period covered by the search and keywords used in searching. Details of articles found in the search but excluded later should be given. This may include reasons associated with irrelevance of work to the subject of the review or low quality.

The results section summarises the main findings reported in the articles reviewed. One useful way of presenting results from many studies is in table form (Table 2.3).

**Table 2.3**  Compliance of insulin use by diabetics (fictitious reports and data)

| Article | No. of patients | Age range of patients (mean) | Method of measuring compliance | No. (%) of patients compliant |
|---|---|---|---|---|
| Smith (1987) | 50 | 50–65 (55) | Self-report | 42 (84) |
| Jones (1992) | 56 | 55–75 (62) | Self-report | 48 (86) |
| Brown (1995) | 55 | 57–70 (62) | Blood sugar level | 28 (51) |

The table should be accompanied by text highlighting key points you wish to make about the data. This may include areas of agreement or disagreement between studies, and comments on any of the methods used by the researchers in obtaining their results.

The review ends with a discussion of your findings and any conclusions you wish to make. This may highlight important gaps in the field or how research in the area could be taken forward, including implications for healthcare practice.

## Summary

Compiling a literature review is a crucial part of the research process. The first task is to search the literature for articles on your particular subject of interest. This is aided by the use of a range of bibliographic tools such as indexing journals. The collection of articles must then be assessed for relevance and quality. Finally, the whole process should be documented in the form of a structured report. The whole endeavour requires certain skills, planning, time and access to good library facilities. However, a good review will provide an overview of the research already conducted, identify gaps or limitations in the research and act as a sounding board for future research ideas.

*Exercise 4*

Summarising your results.

1.  Scan the list of references from the previous exercise. Use title or abstract information to assess the relevance of each one. Make a note of relevant articles.

2.    Collect together copies of the relevant articles from your library.
3.    Extract key information from each relevant article and enter in a table (see Table 2.3 for an example).

# Answers to exercises

Since the exercises for this chapter are to a large extent based on self-selected examples, it is not feasible to provide specific answers to the exercises. You should, however, draw on the guidelines provided in the text when approaching them.

# References

Crombie I K (1996) *The Pocket Guide to Critical Appraisal*. BMJ Publishing Group, London.

Fletcher A, Cullum N and Sheldon T A (1997) A systematic review of compression treatment for venous leg ulcers. *British Medical Journal*. **315**: 576–80.

Hallam L (1994) Primary medical care outside normal working hours: review of published work. *British Medical Journal*. **308**: 249–53.

Liu D, Wettergren M, Lins P E and Adamson U (1990) Combined insulin–glibenclamide therapy of NIDDM patients in primary healthcare. A follow-up study of its compliance and efficacy and a review of the literature. *Scandinavian Journal of Primary Health Care*. **8**(4): 213–17.

Roberts I, Kramer M S and Suissa S (1996) Does routine visiting prevent childhood injury? A systematic review of randomised controlled trials. *British Medical Journal*. **312**: 29–33.

Weinberg H (1990) Asthma in primary care patients: challenges and controversies. *Postgraduate Medicine*. **88**(5): 107–10, 113–14.

Wood J (1991) A review of antenatal care initiatives in primary care settings. *British Journal of General Practice*. **41**(342): 26–30.

# Further reading

Livesey B and Strickland-Hodge B (1989) *How to Search the Medical Sources*. Gower, Aldershot.

Stickland-Hodge B (1986) *How to Use Index Medicus and Excerpta Medica*. Gower, Aldershot.

Warren K S (ed.) (1981) *Coping with the Biomedical Literature: A Primer for the Scientist and Clinician*. Praeger, New York.

# CHAPTER THREE

# Ethical considerations in research

*Nigel Mathers, Amanda Howe and Amanda Hunn*

## Introduction

Before you can embark on carrying out health services research with patients, you are likely to require ethical approval. You may wonder why all this bureaucracy is needed. But history shows us that prior to the development of ethical and human rights over the last 40 years, patients' rights were often ignored and, indeed, many individuals were seriously harmed by medical experimentation.

In the UK today, ethical standards are enforced by a national framework of local research ethics committees (LRECs) in combination with a set of regional multicentre research ethics committees (MRECs). These committees operate to:

- protect the patient/subjects
- protect the patient's rights
- provide the general public with reassurance.

Each committee is made up of eight to 18 members, some of whom will have clinical responsibility and research experience. There must be a minimum of one GP, one nurse and one lay person. The function of the REC is to address issues such as:

- informed patient consent
- coercion of research subjects
- confidentiality
- privacy
- the potential damage or threat to the patient
- how will the research benefit society.

These issues are based on theories and principles which are outlined in more detail later.

Ethical decisions in research are also subject to the dictates of *scientific validity*. It is our belief that poor-quality research is an ethical issue and, indeed, this is also the case with many LRECs to whom you will be submitting your research proposals if you wish to research on human subjects. If a scientific study is fundamentally flawed or guidelines on good clinical practice have not been followed then this is an ethical issue since one is asking, as the researcher, for cooperation in a study which is unlikely to yield useful results.

## Working through this chapter

In addition to the written text, this chapter includes exercises with practical work on observation and note taking. It is suggested that as you work through the chapter, you establish for yourself a 'reflective log', linking the work in the chapter to your own research interests and needs, and your reflections on ethical issues in your own research.

Having successfully completed this chapter, you should:

* know the principles on which ethical decisions are based
* be able to apply these principles to your own research
* be able to describe the processes required to obtain informed consent
* make an application for ethical approval to your local research ethics committee or a multicentre research ethics committee (whichever is most appropriate).

# Why we need ethical approval

Preparing to seek ethical approval may seem like an awful lot of work, but it is important to remember some of the terrible crimes that have been committed against humanity in the name of medical research, and to understand that rules governing ethics in medical research are there for a good reason. Everyone knows about the atrocities committed during the Second World War in Nazi Germany which led to the establishment of the 1947 Nuremberg Code of Practice and in turn the 1964 Declaration of Helsinki. However, few people are aware of some of the unethical activities which have passed as research in more recent times.

One of the most infamous studies is the Tuskegee Syphilis Study. In 1932, a study of 600 black men was undertaken in the USA. The hidden aim was to study the long-term effects of untreated syphilis. Four hundred of the men with the disease were never told of their infection and were never treated despite the fact that treatment became available. The study was not brought to an end until the 1970s. As recently as the 1980s, a study was carried out in New Zealand to examine the natural progression of carcinoma of the cervix. Conventional treatment was withheld from women in the trial and the women were not asked for their consent.

Ultimately, many of the ethical problems arising from these studies are concerned with the issue of 'informed consent'. Occasionally, studies are carried out and given ethical approval even though informed consent has not been sought, because to do so would influence the outcome of the trial (Smith 1997). This is a debatable point and, indeed, there is pressure on journals not to publish research findings if informed consent has not been sought.

# Ethical principles

Before discussing the practical aspects of gaining ethical approval, it is important to understand some of the theoretical issues that underlie ethics in health services research. There are three main approaches that underpin all of our ethical thinking about research.

The first main approach to ethical thinking is the goal-based approach. Based on the consequentialist theory, the approach assumes that we should try and produce the greatest possible balance of value over disvalue. A researcher taking this approach would believe that if the intended outcome of the research is worthwhile then the means to achieving that outcome is worthwhile. This implies that discomfort to one individual may be justified by the consequences for society as a whole. However, even if the research itself is very ethical, it is of no use if the outcome is of little value, so the outcome is as important as the process.

The second approach is duty based. Your duty as a researcher is founded on your own set of moral principles. As a researcher you will have a duty to yourself and to the individual who is participating in the research. So even if the outcome of the proposed research is for a good cause, if it involves the researcher lying or deceiving his subjects in some way then this would be regarded as unethical.

The rights-based approach takes a similar perspective to the duty-based approach. The rights of the individual are assumed to be all-important, thus a subject's right to refuse must be upheld whatever the consequences for the research. This is based on the idea that we should always follow natural laws and rights. This means that our ethical responsibilities are primarily to the individual and that every human being, including yourself, should be respected even if this may have some unfortunate consequences. This is one of the key aspects of the 'doctor–patient relationship'.

It is important to realise that two researchers may come to different conclusions but both may have acted ethically. This is because some of the principles which are derived from these approaches may be in conflict and, depending on which approach one subscribes to, some principles rate higher than others in order of importance. These four principles are outlined below.

The principles are derived from the ethical approaches outlined above. They are always binding unless they are in conflict with other principles, in which case it is necessary to justify why one principle has been chosen over the other. This is the basis for moral reasoning.

# Autonomy

*Autonomy – we ought to respect the right to self-determination*

The first principle is autonomy. Our duty as researchers is both to recognise someone's capacities and perspectives and their right to make choices about whether or not they take part in any research project. We also need to treat that person so as to allow them to act in an autonomous way. In research, autonomy is protected by ensuring that any consent to participate in the study is informed or 'real'. This means that it is not enough to explain something about your project to a particular subject, it is the understanding and free choice whether or not to participate that is the key issue. There must be no coercion of any sort, either direct or indirect, to participate in a particular research project. For example, paying a subject a relatively large sum of money to participate in a study can be construed as coercion. This is because a subject on a low income may have less choice than someone on a higher income whether or not to take part. Similarly, flattering children by telling them their parents would approve of them taking part in your study to 'help other people' could also be considered a form of coercion.

# Non-maleficence

*Non-maleficence – we ought not to inflict evil or harm*

This principle states that we may not inflict harm on, or expose, people to unnecessary risk as a result of our research project. This is particularly important if our subjects may not be competent in some way, such as having the ability to give informed consent. It is not an absolute principle like autonomy, but it is clearly important if, for example, we wish to perform some invasive procedure as part of our research which may not benefit the subject and put him or her at some risk of harm.

In medicine, non-maleficence obliges doctors to provide treatment and keep people alive. However, this obligation to treat may be over-ridden when (a) the treatment is pointless with no prospect of improvement, or (b) when the side-effects of a particular treatment compromise the patient's quality of life. The recent example of 'Child B' with leukaemia is a case in point.

The family is usually thought to have priority in making decisions about treatment where the person is thought not to be competent to make that decision for themselves. This of course is in conflict with the principle of autonomy. However, the obligation of the doctor is to help the family become adequate decision makers by providing a supportive environment for discussion and sufficient information to make choices.

# Beneficence

*Beneficence – we ought to further others' legitimate interests*

This is the principle that obliges us to take positive steps to help others to pursue their interests. These interests clearly have to be legitimate. It is the basis and justification for the actions of all health professions, but there are limits as with autonomy and non-maleficence. For example, there may be a conflict between the principle of autonomy (the right of a person to make a free and informed choice as to whether or not to take part in the study) and beneficence (where part of the study involves non-disclosure of medical information to that person since it may do them harm). Paternalism occurs when a researcher acts on the belief that an individual's views should be disregarded since it is in society's interest to do so. Say, for example, I am pursuing my study on wheezy children and urban air pollution. I find that one of the children who had agreed to take part in the study not only has asthma but also a degenerative lung disease. The child herself may not be aware of this diagnosis and it may not be in the child's interest to inform her of the diagnosis. Should this, though, be the role of the researcher? Here the two principles of autonomy and beneficence are in conflict. If one principle were to be over-ridden by another then we must be able to justify that decision. There would have to be some evidence that paternalism would, on balance, provide greater benefit than autonomy. For those who are interested, this decision would be based on a utilitarian theory.

# Justice

*Justice – we ought to ensure fair entitlement to resources*

This principle is concerned with people receiving their due. This means that people should be treated equally in every way since not all people are equally competent or equally healthy. An example of this in the research study would be that an individual from an ethnic minority should have an equal opportunity to participate in a particular study as everyone else. If I am enrolling children into my study of asthma and urban air pollution then all children should have an equal chance of taking part. This is particularly the case if, on the basis of the study, new treatment was to be offered. It may be necessary therefore to translate questionnaires into other languages.

Proxy decision making is when a decision is made by someone other than the individual directly involved when he or she is not competent to choose or refuse. If a mother is making a decision on behalf of her daughter whether to participate in a study, she may do this by acting in the child's 'best interest' if the child is not competent to give her consent.

# Ethical rules

The ethical rules of research, like principles, are not absolute in that one may over-ride another, although clearly this must be justified. These rules are essential for the development of trust between researchers and study participants. Like the ethical principles on which the rules are based, there are four.

## Veracity

All subjects in any research project should always be told the truth. There is no justification for lying, but this is not the same as non-disclosure of information should it, in particular, invalidate the research.

## Privacy

When subjects enrol in a research study they grant access to themselves, but this is not unlimited access. Access is a broad term and generally includes viewing, touching or having information about them. If someone has agreed to participate in a research study then this does not give the researcher automatic access to their medical records. *Informed consent* for the collection of data from individual medical records can only be given at the outset of the study.

'Informed consent' is the term associated with research of human subjects and is concerned with the extent to which prospective participants are made aware of the exact nature of the research and their right to agree or decline to participate.

## Confidentiality

Although someone may grant limited access to him or herself they may not relinquish control over any information obtained. Certainly, no information obtained with the patient's or subject's permission from their medical records should be disclosed to any third person without that individual's consent. This applies not only to written records but also conversations. Confidentiality can therefore be violated if one talks about one's subjects in the pub, for example, or if their medical records or research records are left in a public place by mistake so that others can read them.

However, confidentiality can be over-ridden by the obligation to fulfil another obligation. For example, in the course of a study I find out that a child's mother has recently attempted suicide and has told no one. In this instance, I as a researcher have an obligation to over-ride the rule of confidentiality and intervene on the mother's behalf by informing a relevant health professional.

## Fidelity

Fidelity means keeping our promises and avoiding negligence with information (as above). If we agree, for example, to send a summary of our research findings to participants in a study we should do so. It is a particular problem when clinical research is being done since although the clinical role is primarily concerned with the patient's welfare, a research project may be for society's benefit not the patient's.

# How to obtain patients' consent

Gaining informed consent from a patient is an essential part of any research. The key point to bear in mind is that the patient is able to make an informed choice about his or her role in the research.

## Study design

Before recruiting patients to a study it is essential that you consider the design of the study and ensure that it is ethical. For example, does the study really need a control arm? Is the sample size sufficient to show a difference? Is the sample size unnecessarily large?

Once you have decided to embark on the study design of your choice you need to decide how patients will be selected for inclusion in the trial and at what stage in the process you will seek their informed consent. It may be important to consider the 'healthy volunteer effect' where the very fact of volunteering for a study makes the subjects unrepresentative of the rest of the population.

If your proposed study includes a *control* arm or a group receiving some sort of *placebo* treatment, then you must still seek informed consent from this group. Just because they are receiving normal treatment, this does not exclude them from the same rights as those subjects receiving the experimental intervention.

## What patients need to know

Patients need to be told not only about the study but also about other options if they decide not to participate. If they agree to participate patients should be informed of their chances of receiving placebo treatment as opposed to an intervention of some kind. They also need to know about all the possible risks.

# Written information and consent

Informed consent should always be sought in writing, preferably using a consent form (see p. 66). A copy of the form should also be given to the patient. It is vital that the patient should also understand that they have the right to withdraw from the study at any stage, and they may need an initial cooling-off period whilst they think about the study.

It is important to give any information in a written form, since some people may find it difficult to take in all the information verbally and probably need time to reflect on the study and what it involves. Any written material given to the patient should be written in plain English using easily understood lay terms. Medical jargon should be avoided. For instance, the average lay person would not understand the term 'myocardial infarction'. It is therefore important to try and use alternative lay terms wherever possible. It helps if the material is written in short sentences and is typed in a large typeface. It may be difficult to judge how easy the material is to read, especially when you are very close to the subject area and used to the clinical terminology. It is possible to assess the reading age of your written material using various tests such as the 'Fog Index' or the 'Flesch Reading Ease Score' (see the Glossary for further information). Obviously written material for ethnic minorities should be translated into the appropriate languages.

# Setting and timing

The setting and timing when seeking informed consent is obviously crucial. It is important that patients do not feel pressurised into agreeing to the study. There needs to be sufficient time to take in the information and to discuss the study and ask questions. Immediately after a serious diagnosis is not usually a good time, since patients may need time to reflect on their condition and may not take in any other information. Subjects must also be given sufficient time to think about the study before committing themselves. There is some evidence that patients with impaired cognitive functioning are better able to function when giving consent in their own home as opposed to a clinical setting.

# Vulnerable subjects

Special care needs to be taken when seeking informed consent from children, the elderly, those who are mentally impaired or those who may be vulnerable to coercion. In the case of children, additional consent will need to be sought from the parents and in the case of the elderly, consent from relatives or carers may also be necessary. However, consent by proxy is open to abuse and it is particularly important to explain all the possible risks and discomfort which may be suffered to a third person. Witnessed consent may also be useful when seeking consent from the infirm.

Whilst parents can give proxy consent on behalf of their children, if the child is deemed to be sufficiently mature then the consent of a parent is not required. Likewise, parental consent cannot over-ride a child's refusal to participate.

The issue of proxy consent is a very difficult one and the simple answer is to try to avoid doing research which includes vulnerable subjects wherever possible. Only if the research to be undertaken could be of potential benefit to the subjects involved and can only be done in that particular group, should vulnerable subjects be included in a study.

# Approaching a local research ethics committee

## In what circumstances do you need ethical approval?

If you are going to recruit patients into a study via healthcare professionals or institutions, or if a third party such as a researcher is going to gain access to confidential medical records or tissue samples, then you will almost certainly need to gain ethical approval. Ethics committees in different areas tend to have different requirements, so it may be best to check with your local ethics committee to see what their requirements are. Remember, however, there are other ways of recruiting patients, apart from using NHS records. For instance, if you were to recruit your respondents directly from a self-help group or stop people in the street with a particular condition, then you might not need to apply for ethical approval depending upon the type of research you are proposing to do. It is dangerous to assume that you don't need ethical approval and if you are in any doubt it is advisable to approach the Chair of your local research ethics committee to check first.

## What do ethics committees want to know?

Clearly, when writing a submission for a research proposal to the local research ethics committee, one needs to bear in mind the four key principles and the four rules of ethical research outlined above. These rules and principles justify all of our specific actions and judgements when doing research. Researchers, when asking for approval for their studies, should in the first instance approach the Secretary of the local research ethics committee (LREC) and discuss the requirements of the committee. These will normally include a fairly detailed pro forma, which needs to be completed and submitted to all members of the committee prior to the researchers' appearance before that committee. Various practical aspects of the research will normally be enquired about, such as the arrangements for indemnity should anything go wrong and the licensing of a particular medication. Whilst one needs to meet the requirements of the ethical principles and rules, it is also important to bear in mind the scientific aspects of the study, such as research design.

Poorly designed research is also considered by many people to be unethical. Researchers should not be surprised if questions are directed towards some scientific aspects of the study since, as stated in the introduction, validity is an important component of ethical review. One of the questions often asked concerns the power of the study. Consulting a statistician prior to submission could be very helpful.

Remember the key questions that the ethics committee will be asking are:

- Is the research valid?
  - How important is the research question?
  - Can the question be answered?
- Is the welfare of the research subject under threat?
  - What will participating involve?
  - Are the risks necessary and acceptable?
- Is the dignity of the research subject upheld?
  - Will consent be sought?
  - Will confidentiality be respected?

## What happens if my research covers more than one area?

For those researchers planning to carry out large-scale studies which will fall into the boundaries of five or more local research ethics committees, ethical permission should be sought in a single application from a multicentre research ethics committee (MREC), rather than approaching each separate LREC.

If you are planning to do a national study or propose to sample your subjects from more than one region, you only need to gain approval from one MREC. A single MREC can give approval from studies covering the whole country. Once approval has been given by a MREC you will still need to inform each local REC, but they can only accept or reject the study or make change to the patient information sheet for local reasons. The LREC cannot substantially amend a protocol which has been approved by a MREC. Although each region has its own MREC, you need only approach your local MREC in your region for a multisite study.

*Exercise 1*

Which of the three ethical approaches described at the beginning of this chapter are addressed in the following areas:

- validity of the research
- welfare of the research subject
- dignity of the research subject.

Answers to this question are given at the end of this chapter.

# Ethical conduct

Having carefully designed your study and obtained ethical approval, you now start to collect and analyse data. There are numerous examples in the scientific literature of authors behaving unethically during the process of doing their research. There is a spectrum of inadvertent error through to outright fraud. There may be scientific errors such as inappropriate and inadequate observations, poor-quality data analysis and selective quotes from references. Further along this spectrum there may be substantial bias in the selection of the sample or frank abuse of statistics.

Gift authorship may also be considered an example of scientific misconduct whereby favours are returned in kind by including one's partner, supervisor or professional colleague on a publication as a reward even though they have made no substantial contribution to the paper. Salami publication is also thought to be a form of scientific misconduct whereby the same piece of work is simply sliced and repeatedly published in different journals with differing emphases. Further along this spectrum towards outright fraud, activities such as manipulating data or suppressing inconvenient data should be included as well as an undeclared interest in the outcome such as pressure from a pharmaceutical company to produce a 'good result' for their drug for which the researcher receives a 'bonus'. Finally, at the extreme end of this spectrum outright fraud may indeed take place and this would include plagiarism of other people's original work or, indeed, piracy of their results.

# Summary

The main points made in this chapter are that ethical decisions are based on three main approaches: duty, rights and goal based. Research studies should be judged ethically on three sets of criteria, namely: ethical principles, ethical rules and also scientific criteria. The latter is often neglected but is important since if a study design is poor or the sample size insufficient then the study is not capable of demonstrating anything and consequently could be regarded as unethical.

The four key ethical principles are:

*   autonomy
*   non-maleficence
*   beneficence
*   justice.

The four key ethical rules are:

*   veracity
*   privacy
*   confidentiality
*   fidelity.

The chapter has also provided guidance on how ethical approval may be obtained for research studies in primary care.

## Exercise 2

Read the following research proposal in which a researcher wishes to recruit carers of patients with chronic severe arthritis. The main aim of the study is to examine carer satisfaction with primary healthcare and social services.

1.  If you were a member of a local research ethics committee, how would you use the previously considered rules and principles to decide whether or not to give this study ethical approval?
2.  Make suggestions as to how the ethical aspects of this protocol might be made more successful.

Answers to the exercise are given at the end of this chapter.

# The protocol

## Title

What are the needs of those caring for patients with severe arthritis in the community?

## Research investigators

Dr Jane White, Senior Registrar, Rheumatology Department, St. Anywhere's
Sister Liz Brown, Senior Nursing Officer, Community Health Trust, Ipsbit
James Black, Senior Social Worker, Social Services, Ipsbit District Council
(Correspondence to Dr White)

## Main aims of the study

To elucidate the views of informal carers for patients with severe arthritis on the services offered by community and social services.

# Potential value of the study

The main outcomes of the study are to inform the subsequent health and social services delivered to patients in this category, and to enhance carer satisfaction.

## Background and summary of the literature

Arthritis is a major cause of disability and poor quality of life, especially in older patients. It accounts for 20% of all those over the age of 65 who are housebound and chronically dependent on others for their physical care. Although it is common, little is known about the perceived needs of those suffering from severe arthritis, and less still about how this affects their carers. Lynson's survey asked community nurses for their assessment of the clinical needs of arthritics, but the assessments were not standardised, and the information gained had a clinical bias. Multiple pathology and interacting social factors make the picture more complex: many arthritics will not be housebound due to arthritis alone, and increased disposable income may increase mobility due to the purchasing of aids or drivers. There is, therefore, a need to gain a more detailed picture of the detailed reasons why sufferers from severe arthritis of any causation become effectively 'housebound' and to assess how scarce resources can be used most effectively and efficiently to improve quality of life.

## Method

Thirty carers will be sought for interview by contacting the GPs of patients known to either the community trust or the department of rheumatology. GPs will be asked to confirm that the patient concerned suffers from severe arthritis, that there is no reason not to contact the family and to give details of those in the same household who are likely to be the main carers. The letters will then be sent to those persons, and all those willing will be visited by a member of the research team at home to carry out a detailed semi-structured interview (schedule and letters attached). This will occur once only and will last about 30 minutes. Those consenting to be interviewed will be asked to agree to tape recording of the interview for ease of transcription. Data derived from interviews will be stored in Dr White's office.

## Sample size and data analysis

Thirty interviews is considered a large sample in qualitative studies. The data will be analysed according to Glaser and Strauss's 'grounded theory' approach which allows key themes to emerge from the data, thus avoiding bias by the researchers. Transcribed data will be analysed using 'Nudist' computer software.

## Site of the study

Carers' homes, or at the clinic or GP surgery if they prefer.

## Duration of study

Six months, from January to June 1998.

## Potential hazards to subjects

None.

### Procedures of discomfort

None.

### Sponsorship

Pens for GPs kindly donated by the Arthritis Council.

### Compensation to subjects

None (free pen to general practitioners if patient reply slip returned).

### Access to data

- Only by research team.
- Paper data will be destroyed at the end of the study.

### Enclosures

- Cover letter for research subjects (Box 3.1).
- Information sheet for research subjects (Box 3.2).

---

**Box 3.1**    Cover letter for research subjects

Dr J. White<br>
Senior Registrar<br>
Rheumatology Department<br>
St Anywhere's<br>
Grey St.<br>
Gladwell

Dear _____ ,

'Study of the needs of those caring for patients with severe arthritis in the community'

Your name has been passed to us by your family doctor, Dr _____. We understand that your relation, _____, suffers from severe arthritis. We are therefore writing to you to ask whether you might be willing to help us with an important study into the problems which you and your relative or friend face due to their health problems. The attached sheet explains more about what we are trying to do and how you might be able to help us. When you have read it carefully, please return the reply-slip below in the prepaid envelope saying whether we can contact you again about the study. If you have any questions before making a decision, you are very welcome to phone me on 0137 542345 (9 a.m.–6 p.m.).

With thanks for your time and consideration.

Dr Jane White

---

**Box 3.2**    Information sheet for research subjects

*Study of the needs of those caring for patients with severe arthritis in the community*

*What is the study about?*
Arthritis is a major cause of disability and poor quality of life, especially in older patients. It accounts for 20% of all those over the age of 65 who are housebound and chronically dependent on others for their physical care. Although it is common, little is known about the perceived needs of those suffering from severe arthritis, and less still about how this affects their carers. There is a need to gain a more detailed picture of the reasons why sufferers from severe arthritis of any causation become effectively 'housebound' and to assess how scarce resources can be used most effectively and efficiently to improve quality of life. We hope that the study will improve services to families such as yours. The local ethics committee has supported this study.

*Who is involved in the study?*
The study is being carried out by members of the Rheumatology Department, St Anywhere's, the Community Health Trust, Ipsbit and Social Services, Ipsbit District Council.

   The people being interviewed have been identified by NHS staff at the hospital and in the community who know your relative with arthritis through being their doctor or nurse. Your GP has confirmed that your relative is in this group, and that you are their main carer.

*Do I have to take part?*
No. The study is entirely optional. If you choose not to be involved, this will not affect your care or that of your relative in any way.

*What is involved?*
If you are willing to allow us to, one of our research team will telephone you to make an appointment to visit at home (or at the clinic if you prefer). They would like about 45 minutes to ask you some questions about your experiences. They will tape-record your comments if this is acceptable, in order to help them make an accurate record of your comments.

*What happens to the information?*
All information you give is entirely confidential. The tape recordings are transcribed into written words, and all the comments analysed together to give us a full picture of your experiences and others like you. The data is kept in a locked office at the hospital and only the research team can see it. At the end of the study all original material will be destroyed.

*What if I wish to complain?*
Please raise any queries or difficulties with a member of the research team. If you want to telephone, please contact Dr White on 0137 542345 (9 a.m.–6 p.m. weekdays). If you have major cause for complaint, please contact the Patient Relations Officer at St. Anywhere's who are responsible for insuring this study.

*Now please complete the consent form.*

**Box 3.3**    Consent form for research subjects

Have you read the information provided?                                    Yes/No

Have you received enough information about the study?                      Yes/No

Do you understand that you can withdraw from the study:

*   at any time
*   without having to give any reason
*   without affecting your future medical care or that of your relatives?   Yes/No

Do you agree to take part in this study?                                   Yes/No

Signed _____          Date _____
(Research subject)

*   Consent form for research subjects (Box 3.3).
*   GP letter (Box 3.4).
*   Information slip (Box 3.5).

**Box 3.4**    GP letter

> Dr J. White
> Senior Registrar
> Rheumatology Department
> St Anywhere's
> Grey St.
> Gladwell

Dear Dr _____ ,

'Study of the needs of those caring for patients with severe arthritis in the community'

Your name has been passed to us by _____ . We understand that you have a patient, _____, who suffers from severe arthritis. We are therefore writing to you to ask whether you might be willing to help us with an important study into the problems which your patient and their carers face due to their health problems. The attached sheet explains more about what we are trying to do and how they might be able to help us. We would be very grateful if, before we contact them, you could spend a few moments completing the slip below to ensure that it is appropriate to contact them, and that we have their correct address. In return, we enclose a pen as a token of our appreciation for your time and trouble.

With thanks,

Dr J. White

---

**Box 3.5**    Information slip

Patient _____

Address _____

_____

_____

_____

Name of main carer known to you  _____

Address _____

_____

_____

Is this person your patient? _____

Do you in your knowledge of their situation think it is OK to contact this household?

_____

_____

_____

*Thank you. Now please return this slip in the prepaid envelope.*

---

# Answers to exercises

## Exercise 1

1.    Validity of the research addresses the goal-based approach.
2.    Welfare of the research subject addresses the duty-based approach.
3.    Dignity of the research subject addresses the rights-based approach.

## Exercise 2

The kinds of issues a local research committee might raise about this protocol include:

### Scientific validity

Are the identifiers for the patient group really clear? 'Arthritis' and 'housebound' are rather vague and overinclusive categories.

Are the aims and objectives of this study really clear enough to yield a useful result? In particular, the researchers seem constantly to confuse the information they require about carers' perceptions with those likely to come from the patients themselves.

Is the value of qualitative studies such as these sufficiently great to justify the resources that will go into it?

### Confidentiality

The professional carers (hospital or community staff) do not have the permission of the patient to release their details to the research team. Similarly, the general practitioner has no permission from either carer or patient to pass on or confirm details to the researchers. The patient's permission should be sought in the first instance by the professional staff directly, and the patient should then opt to allow the research team to enter a further dialogue with them directly. The privacy of the carer is also an issue.

### Practicalities

The staff involved may not take the trouble to carry out the requests.

The general practitioners may not have the information they require about the carers.

### Coercion

The information given states repeatedly what an important study this is, and also that the ethics committee approve this. The researchers should not claim or imply benefit from the study as they do not know what the outcome of the data collection will be.

The implication that the professional carers have seen fit to release their details may make some patients and their carers feel they must conform and join in the study.

### Principles

The main problems here seem to be with:

*   autonomy (various assumptions are made about the rights of the researchers to get access to personal information – *confidentiality* and *privacy*)

- beneficence (will the study do any good given its lack of *scientific validity* and *potential bias?*)
- justice (a small point might be made about why the general practitioner gets a gift but not the lay participants).

### Alternatives

- Clear objectives are needed. This is possible even in qualitative studies.
- Information should be requested on how evidence from this study will influence social services offered: there should be some potential for change if this is to be of value.
- The patient group should be identified more clearly or more direct access to carers should be obtained.
- Professionals should be asked to give the letters out, so patients only reply if they are willing to participate.
- Patients should be asked to give details to carers, so that again they are not identified to the researchers unless they are willing for this to occur.
- The value of the study and its support from local ethics committees should not be stressed.

# References

Smith R (1997) Informed consent: the intricacies. *British Medical Journal.* **314**: 1059–60.

# Further reading

Beauchamp T and Childres J (1989) *Principles of Biomedical Ethics.* Oxford University Press, Oxford.

Evans D and Evans M (1996) *A Decent Proposal.* John Wiley, Chichester.

Lock S and Wells F (1996) *Fraud and Misconduct in Medical Research.* BMJ Publications, London.

Royal College of Nursing Research Advisory Group (1993) *Ethics Related to Research in Nursing.* Scutari Press, Harrow.

Royal College of Physicians of London (1992) Guidelines on good practice of ethics committees in medical research for human subjects. *Journal of the Royal College of Physicians.* **26**: 292.

Social Research Association (1995) *Social Research Association Ethical Guidelines.* Thompson Press, London.

Tranter J (1997) The patient's rights in clinical research. *Professional Nurse.* **12**: 335–7.

Wager E, Tooley P, Emanuel M *et al.* (1995) Get patients' consent to enter clinical trials. *British Medical Journal.* **311**: 734–7.

# CHAPTER FOUR

# Health needs assessment

*Linda East, Vicky Hammersley and Beverley Hancock*

## Introduction

The purpose of this chapter is to introduce readers to health needs assessment in contemporary primary healthcare. It has been written at an exciting time, when the mechanisms are being set in motion which will make health services increasingly primary care led. The NHS (Primary Care) Act of 1997 will encourage new ways of working and increased flexibility in service delivery. The following quotation is taken from *Primary Care: Delivering the Future*, the Government White Paper which underpins the new legislation:

> 'Primary care depends on the contribution of a wide range of professionals working together to meet the needs of all patients in the community. At its heart is the family doctor and the general practice team of nurses, managers and, increasingly, other professionals. They need to work closely with community nurses, midwives and therapists to offer comprehensive and appropriate support to their patients. But primary care does not stop here – pharmacists, dentists and optometrists on the high street provide essential services as, for example, do social workers and housing officers from local authorities. The proposals in this document should enable all of these to play their part better, to extend their role where appropriate and to ensure that services are coordinated around the needs of individuals.'
> [Department of Health 1996, p. 4]

The last sentence, in particular, is highly relevant to the purpose of this chapter when it states that services should be 'coordinated around the needs of individuals'. Healthcare usually takes the individual as its starting point, but primary care is also informed by a public health ethos which concerns the health and welfare of people in groups. Primary care practitioners do not assess individuals in isolation from the communities in which they live. They recognise that the health experiences of individuals are affected by whether they reside in towns or disadvantaged inner-cities, in isolated farm houses or sprawling council estates. Primary care practitioners know about the range of local services and facilities and are part of local networks of formal and informal care.

Primary care practitioners serve other communities as well as those based on shared residence of a particular location. Within the neighbourhood there will be institutions such as schools and factories where people have health needs. There may also be groups of people whose needs reflect the social and physiological legacies of their ethnic origins, or who are drawn to the area by particular facilities, from women's refuges to universities. People who once would have lived their lives in institutions now make their homes in more or less supported environments in the community, and therefore need improved access to the services of primary care.

Primary care workers need to know how to assess individuals, how to manage their care and how to encourage healthier lifestyles. They require a great understanding of people's ways of life and the health problems they experience and they need to know how to use this understanding to systematically assess the needs of people in groups. Health needs assessment aims to achieve health gain for groups by identifying need and effectively targeting resources. The process of health needs assessment takes the locality as its starting point, a point recognised by the Department of Health (1996, p. 4):

> 'Our aim is to enable local people to shape and develop high-quality primary healthcare services in a way which makes best use of the resources available and best suits local circumstances and needs.'

Health needs assessment means identifying local strengths as well as difficulties, and devising strategies which build on the former and minimise the latter. This chapter is dedicated to helping primary care practitioners understand the principles of health needs assessment. The following sections will:

- introduce the reader to different approaches to health needs assessment
- identify appropriate methods for collecting information
- discuss how this information can be interpreted and applied in practice.

After using this chapter, the reader will be able to:

- discuss the role and functions of health needs assessment in contemporary primary healthcare
- outline four key approaches to health needs assessment (the practice profile, the community profile, the life-cycle framework and the group of special interest)
- identify methods of collecting quantitative information from public and patient records and epidemiological data
- analyse the scope and appropriateness of four approaches to primary data collection (observation, surveys, qualitative interviews and focus groups)
- consider ways in which the results of health needs assessment can be used in primary healthcare practice.

# Defining health needs assessment

It is difficult to offer a concise definition of health needs assessment because of the debates which surround the concepts of 'health' and 'need'. Economists, in particular, are sceptical of the whole idea of need, preferring to think in terms of demand and supply. Primary healthcare practitioners use this debate to ask: What do people *need* to maintain a worthwhile quality of life? Most people would acknowledge that adequate food and heating are essentials – but do families really *need* a television or a washing machine? Readers interested in following up this theoretical debate are referred to the work of Doyal and Gough (1991), who argue that there *are* basic human needs and also intermediate needs crucial to the universal goal of full participation in society. Ultimately, everyone wants to avoid harm and be part of society to the degree that they themselves choose. Basic and intermediate needs are the preconditions which must be satisfied before this goal can be realised, as outlined in Box 4.1.

---

**Box 4.1**   Basic and intermediate human needs

*Universal goal*:
- avoidance of serious harm and minimally disabled social participation

*Basic needs*:
- an optimum level of physical health and 'autonomy of agency' (i.e. freedom to make decisions over one's life)

*Intermediate needs*:
- adequate food and water
- adequate protective housing
- a non-hazardous work environment
- appropriate healthcare
- security in childhood
- significant primary relationships
- physical security
- economic security
- safe birth control and child-bearing
- basic education

From Doyal and Gough (1991).

---

Percy-Smith and Sanderson (1992) used Doyal and Gough's framework to inform a study of local needs in Leeds. They concluded that 'the best way of addressing ill health and the absence of well-being in the longer term, may not be through medical intervention but through measures aimed at alleviating the problems that appear to lead to ill health and lack of well-being' (p. 224). Primary care workers should thus recognise the full range of factors which have the potential to contribute to the overall health profile of a community, and not stick to a narrow medical focus. The Department of Health goes some way towards recognising this when it acknowledges the role of social workers and local authority housing officers in primary care (Department of Health 1996).

## Why carry out health needs assessment?

One rationale for health needs assessment is that of promoting equity in access to a positive state of health and well-being. The philosophy that underpins the principles of *Health for All* emphasises social justice, equity, community participation and responsiveness to the needs of local populations. A second rationale for a research-based approach to health needs assessment lies in the National Health Service reforms that informed the 1991 NHS and Community Care Act. Prior to this, health service planning has been described as supply led, focusing on existing services rather than need and biased towards the acute sector (Pickin and St Leger 1993). Thus, the reforms of the 1990s and the introduction of market principles underpin the second rationale for health needs assessment: to ensure the most clinically efficient and cost-effective distribution of limited resources. Thus, a very different vision of health needs assessment to that enshrined in the principles of *Health for All* emerges, focusing on the need for *healthcare services* as opposed to the need for *health*. It is basically a medical model for healthcare, where need is defined as the presence of a disease which is treatable successfully.

Health authorities and general practitioners seek to purchase care which will achieve both health gain for their populations and the best value for money. There is a danger that preventative work will be marginalised if health need is narrowly defined as the potential for health gain within a disease-focused biomedical framework.

## Who should be involved in health needs assessment?

Under the NHS and Community Care Act (1991), assessment of need within populations is the responsibility of Directors of Public Health working at executive levels within health authorities. Fundholding general practices were charged with a similar responsibility to consider their practice populations and determine spending priorities accordingly. In addition, policies favouring locality management require provider units to take an overview of need in ever smaller and more precise geographical areas.

The concept of the primary healthcare team is expanding to embrace the ideals of working in partnership. The professions traditionally described as 'allied to medicine' all play an essential role in identifying health need, planning, coordinating and delivering care (Department of Health 1996). Nicholas (1996) argues that *every* primary healthcare professional should be able to answer the following questions:

- Do you know the health status of the people for whom you are responsible?
- Do you know how this health status differs from the broader community and district health profiles?

- Is there a need to seek to alter this health status?
- If so, is there a capacity to alter that health status in terms of available knowledge and technology – and of political will?

Assessing health need is important both in terms of promoting health and in determining priorities for resource allocation. The following sections in this chapter will outline some of the techniques primary care workers can use to develop this area of their practice.

# Approaches to health needs assessment

This section will describe four frameworks which can be used to design a health needs assessment project.

It is important that primary healthcare workers have a sound insight into exactly *why* they should carry out a needs assessment. A good way of beginning is to consider some of the questions outlined in Box 4.2.

---

**Box 4.2**    Questions to ask when planning a health needs assessment project

- What is your area of interest which defines the scope of the health need to be addressed? Are you interested in a whole population or a particular subsection such as older people or women?
- What is the size of the problem? How many people share the health need?
- What are the views of patients, carers and the local community? What is known from previous work? Who do you need to talk to locally?
- How do your figures compare with local and national averages? How important is the problem in your practice compared with others?
- What interventions are you already making? Do you have a response to the problem? What are other agencies doing?
- What has worked elsewhere? Is there any relevant literature available or projects which can be visited? Are there examples of 'best practice' in the area you are interested in?
- What could and should you be doing in future? Consider all options, prioritise and develop an action plan.

Adapted from Sheffield Health Authority (1996).

---

The way in which you address these questions will largely depend on the outcome your needs assessment is designed to produce. In this section, we identify four key approaches to the task of assessing health need:

- the practice profile
- the life-cycle framework
- the group of special interest
- the community profile.

These approaches need not be mutually exclusive and the techniques used for gathering information will sometimes overlap. However, thinking about the philosophy which informs each approach will help you to clarify your task.

## The practice profile

The growing importance of primary care in the NHS demands an accurate understanding of what is happening in general practice. The GP contract introduced in 1990 requires practices to submit an annual report to their health authority describing their activities and the population they serve (Ross and Mackenzie 1996). Fundholding practices also need to profile the healthcare needs of their population in order to develop the contracts through which they purchase services.

A recent study undertaken in Nottingham by Muir (1996) reviews the information required to develop a practice profile. Muir's conclusions are summarised in Box 4.3.

---

**Box 4.3**     Information for the practice profile

*Indicators of need*
- Age/sex profile
- Mortality rates
- Socio-economic indicators
- Births

*Indicators of demand*
- GP consultation rates
- Community services contacts
- Standardised admission rates (to secondary care)
- Practice nurse attendances
- Standardised referral rates (to secondary care)
- Waiting-list information

*Resources*
- Staffing levels
- Budget/expenditure

*Outputs*
- Screening/immunisation rates
- Chronic disease management activity rates
- Health promotion activity rates
- Prescribing data

Adapted from Muir (1996).

---

The distinction between need, demand and available resources is important. All these elements are part of needs *assessment* in the practice profile. The indicators used to determine need reflect the population characteristics associated with the burden of ill health. The indicators reflecting demand, on the other hand, give an idea of the services actually used. The profile of resources will describe the means available to meet need and satisfy demand.

It is important to note that the practice profile may fail to capture the dimension of unmet need. It is widely acknowledged that only a small proportion of illness is actually translated into contact with the health services, even in primary care (Ross and Mackenzie 1996). Health needs assessment within the context of a developing practice profile means going beyond current patterns of service usage in order to target need efficiently and effectively. However, the capacity of practices to take up this challenge is inevitably dependent on the human and material resources available.

## The life-cycle framework

This approach was developed by Pickin and St Leger (1993) in an attempt to create a systematic and practical framework for health needs assessment. The human lifespan is divided into nine age bands, for each of which there are key issues associated with health and illness. The life-cycle framework invites the user to consider the wider influences affecting health status at each stage of life, and describes these as 'modifiers'. Pickin and St Leger also discuss the resources available to improve health and identify factors which affect the use of services. Their text could be a useful source of inspiration for any primary healthcare worker who has responsibility for a particular age group and wishes to profile their needs. They follow the structure outlined in Box 4.4 and explore a wide range of issues in relation to health needs assessment at each stage of the lifespan.

---

**Box 4.4**     Structure of the life-cycle framework

| | |
|---|---|
| *Influences on health*: | main influences at each stage of the lifespan, leading causes of morbidity and mortality |
| *Sources of information on health*: | how to access information |
| *Modifiers to health experience*: | socio-economic, environmental, ethnic and cultural influences on health |
| *Health resources*: | subdivided into the individual, the family, the community and formal health services |
| *Modifiers to the use of services*: | socio-economic, environmental, ethnic and cultural influences |
| *Service options*: | discusses ways of extending and improving services for each age group |

Adapted from Pickin and St Leger (1993).

---

Pickin and St Leger suggest their work can be used as a reference which highlights the health issues to consider at each stage of the life cycle and which summarises currently available routine information. They argue that the life-cycle framework can be used to explore health need among groups usually defined in other ways. For example, the needs of 'the homeless' may be very different depending on age, gender and whether or not the homeless adult has dependent children.

## The group of special interest

In approaching the task of health needs assessment, primary care workers may seek to focus on the needs of a particular subgroup of the population. The group selected may be based on age, as outlined above, or may reflect a common characteristic such as gender or ethnic origin. A particularly salient rationale for focusing on a particular group may be because they represent a national priority area as defined in the *Health of the Nation* (Department of Health 1992). Alternatively, groups of special interest may share a particular lifestyle which is the focus of health needs assessment, for example travellers or drug users. For some groups, it may be easy to obtain accurate data, for example women who have recently had babies. For other groups, however, it may be much harder to get an accurate picture as to the numbers involved, for example homeless teenagers on the run from local authority care. In the latter case, sensitive outreach work may be required to accurately profile health need.

An interest in the health needs of a particular group within the practice population is often the starting point for primary healthcare workers enthusiastic to develop the services they provide. For example, a health visitor working in an inner-city neighbourhood was concerned about the well-being of Asian mothers on her case-load. Through interviewing the young women, a range of interventions were identified which enabled the health centre as a whole to improve its services for this particular group of users.

## The community profile

A community profile is defined by Hawtin *et al.* (1994, p. 5) as:

> 'A comprehensive description of the needs of a population that is defined, or defines itself, as a community, and the resources that exist within that community, carried out with the active involvement of the community itself, for the purpose of developing an action plan or other means of improving the quality of life in a community.'

The emphasis in this approach is on members of the public taking an active, and perhaps a leading, role in developing the profile. The sorts of information included in a community profile might include the resources in the area in terms of schools, shops and open space for children to play in. The profile may include looking at crime rates as well as health statistics, and housing conditions as well as high rates of particular diseases. Often residents of a particular area come together to campaign for particular improvements such as traffic calming, and will enlist the help of health professionals to support their case. At other times, it may be the primary healthcare workers who seek to stimulate public awareness of health issues within a neighbourhood, and facilitate the processes of community development. In this case, it will be necessary to adopt a problem-solving, action-oriented approach as described in Box 4.5.

---

**Box 4.5**   Developing a community profile: ten steps

1.   Assembling a group of interested and concerned local people
2.   Initial prioritising of perceived problems
3.   Initial planning and time-scale for the profiling exercise
4.   Mobilising resources – time, money and training for participants in data collection
5.   Gathering data
6.   Analysing data and identifying needs
7.   Presenting results
8.   Taking the profile forward
9.   Working with others
10.  Monitoring and evaluation

Adapted from Burton (1993).

---

Community profiles will vary according to the specific locality and its needs. Whatever the circumstances, the process of producing a profile can be empowering for the group of people involved. It is a good way of building relationships and promoting teamwork between local residents, voluntary groups and public agencies. However, it is important to continue the work once the profile has been completed and to campaign on the needs and problems identified. Primary healthcare workers who take this approach to health needs assessment need a long-term commitment to the neighbourhood and confidence in their own ability to advocate for public health.

## Summary

In approaching health needs assessment it is important to be clear about your purpose – to know what are you trying to find out and to what end. Thinking this through at the beginning will enable you to think more clearly about the kind of information needed, from whom information should be collected and the best way of collecting information. The following sections will explore the sources of evidence for health need in more depth and suggest a variety of strategies which can be applied in primary care.

# Using public health data and patient records

This section will offer practical guidance on how to collect and analyse public and practice-based information and, where relevant, will discuss the strengths and limitations of each data source. The reader is encouraged to undertake the suggested exercises in order to develop insight into quantitative data analysis.

In an ideal world, health needs assessment would be based upon data that describes every individual registered with a general practice or living within a defined neighbourhood. In the real world, this is not possible. The assessment of health need, therefore, will always rely on the analysis and interpretation of existing data. Luckily, a great deal of useful information is routinely available. The available information includes census data and the results of local and national surveys such as the General Household Survey. The *Public Health Common Data Set (PHCDS)* is commissioned by the Department of Health and is presently produced by The National Institute of Epidemiology (University of Surrey, 14 Frederick Sanger Road, Surrey Research Park, Guildford GU2 5YD). The data set was introduced in 1989 as a resource for Directors of Public Health in producing their annual reports, but is now being used for a variety of purposes. The data set has been expanded to include data on morbidity, mortality trends, *Health of the Nation* target indicators and indicators derived from the 1991 census. The *PHCDS* is an annual publication and is distributed to all health authorities. Access to many external data sources (i.e. data collected from outside the practice) can be gained from health authority resource centres, departments of public health, local councils and good public libraries. Data sources described in the following paragraphs comprise demographic data, activity data and health data. These data are usually presented in relation to larger units of a geographically defined population, but can be broken down to the level of a shared postcode.

## Demographic data

Demography refers to the study of populations with reference to the factors which affect it, such as migration and mortality, and the interactions these factors have with social and economic conditions.

### Population data

The choice of population depends on the specific purpose of the health needs assessment exercise. The populations may be as small as an enumeration district (approximately 200 households) but more usually are assessed at the level of the electoral ward or health authority population. For example, a health needs assessment exercise within a general practice may cover all registered patients, whereas a health needs assessment carried out by a health visitor may be limited to all patients on her case-load. Care must be taken when identifying the chosen population as it may overlap several electoral wards, and identifying the characteristics of the total population for comparative purposes may prove difficult. If a practice population is chosen, census information covering each electoral ward can be obtained from the health authority. This includes information about households, as well as individuals, and can be analysed for each variable measured, thus allowing a comparison of all wards covered by the target population for the health needs assessment to be made with local and regional figures. Health authorities can play a positive role in collating and disseminating information.

The age–gender structure of a population, whether it be practice, local or regional, is fundamental to health needs assessment. The baseline population data are derived from the results of the decennial census, and this information can be found in the Office of Population Census and Surveys (OPCS) book entitled *Census 1991 – Key Statistics for Local Authorities*. It is also possible to obtain an age–sex breakdown of a general practice population. Population estimates are calculated by OPCS by taking the census data as a baseline, by using data on births and deaths since the time of the census and then estimating the migration in and out of the district. Population projections refer to educated guesses of population in the future. In carrying out health needs assessment it is important to determine the value of knowing the detailed characteristics of the population, and whether comparison with larger populations is needed. For example, if the assessment is to be used for redistribution of services, then reliable comparisons are essential. If, however, the health needs assessment is to identify the extent of the need for a service within a general practice (e.g. a well man clinic), it is essential to know the extent of the need within the general practice list, but of little interest to compare the extent of the need occurring in a wider population.

## Social characteristics

Most of the information available on the social characteristics of people also comes from *Census 1991*. It analyses the following information for district councils:

- economic activity
- industry of employment
- travel to work
- number of households/household size/economically active adults
- households with children/one-adult households with children
- ethnic group.

A number of the variables collected in the census can be analysed in combination to create indicators for deprivation. There are two widely recognised quantitative measures of deprivation based on the population of electoral wards: the Jarman index and the Townsend score (Box 4.6).

The Jarman index is available at practice level and is the index used to determine extra deprivation payments for general practices. The more positive the Jarman score, the more deprived the community. GPs receive a low-deprivation payment for patients living in wards with an underprivileged area (UPA) score of +30 to +40, medium payments for

---

**Box 4.6** Jarman and Townsend scores

*The Jarman index*

The Jarman underprivileged area (UPA) score is derived from eight census variables:

(1)   % unemployment
(2)   % children under five
(3)   % unskilled workers
(4)   % lone parents
(5)   % pensioners living alone
(6)   % overcrowded households
(7)   % ethnic minority
(8)   % changed address in last year.

A score of 0 is average, and the more positive the score, the more deprived the population.

*The Townsend score*

The Townsend deprivation score is derived from four census variables:

(1)   % households with no car
(2)   % unemployment
(3)   % homes non-owner occupied
(4)   % overcrowded households.

Again, the more positive the Townsend score, the more deprived the population.

---

those wards with a UPA of +40 to +50, and high-deprivation payments in wards with a UPA of more than 50. The score of 0 is average for England and Wales.

There are problems associated with both the Jarman and Townsend scores. Validity is concerned with whether or not an indicator actually measures the underlying attribute which it claims to measure (Robinson and Elkan 1996).

- The Jarman index was initially based on ten variables, and subsequently two have been omitted on grounds of lack of validity.
- In some cases, where direct deprivation is impossible to measure, an appropriate indicator cannot be found.
- Most measures of deprivation rely on the census, and are therefore constrained by the information available in the census.
- The census is decennial, hence information collected and used soon becomes out of date.

As deprivation is closely associated with higher levels of ill health, deprivation indicators are useful proxy measures for health need. Further useful information available in the decennial census includes the number of people who self-report a limiting long-term illness.

The practice database includes the patient's address with postcode, and this information can be used to evaluate the catchment area for the practice, using the ACORN classification (Gillam and Murray 1996). ACORN is an acronym for A Classification Of Residential Neighbourhoods, and is a composite socio-demographic index derived from census variables. The advantage of this method over the Jarman and Townsend indices is that the classification is available at enumeration district level as opposed to electoral ward level. Many electoral wards include pockets of deprivation, such as large estates alongside more affluent neighbourhoods. It is important to identify these areas of deprivation which may be obscured by a low Jarman or Townsend score at ward level.

# Activity data

Information can be collected about the activity of hospitals and health service activity in the community, including general practice. Used in this context, 'activity' means any episode involving contact with patients which is recorded by hand or on computer.

## Hospital in-patient information

From each hospital, a minimum data set for each episode (defined as a period of care received under one hospital consultant) is sent to the Department of Health for collation into national statistics on hospital activity. This includes the specialty of care, diagnosis, admission and discharge date and details about the patient (Unwin *et al.* 1997). The information on diagnosis, coded according to the International Classification of Diseases and/or the type of surgical intervention (OPCS codes), is often regarded as of doubtful accuracy, and activity in private hospitals is not included. A minimum data set system for maternity is also available.

Hospital data are of some use in assessing health need, but their usefulness is limited by problems of lack of data accuracy and completeness and delays in publication (Gillam and Murray 1996). A further problem is that in-patient admission rates are not a proxy for morbidity in the community. A study by Payne *et al.* (1994) showed that only two diseases (respiratory disease and depression) out of the seven diseases or procedures investigated showed a positive correlation between disease prevalence and hospital admission.

Health service indicators are available via the Department of Health, who publish a comparative information package on routine data submissions throughout the NHS. The package compares performance indicators of all provider units and health authorities, and can be obtained from the Department of Health, Room 1418, Euston Tower, 286 Euston Road, London NW1 3DN. Unfortunately, the data are at least 18 months old so should be verified with more recent data before being used to inform significant decisions.

## Community information

The definition of health service activity in the community encompasses the activity of general practitioners and practice-based staff, and of all community health services. Annual practice reports to the health authority could potentially become a very valuable source of data, providing information collected in practice is from a validated, complete database.

Services to the community include:

*   vaccination and immunisation (Korner statistics)
*   family planning services (Korner statistics)
*   maternity and child health services (Korner statistics).

# Health and disease data

In assessing health need, it is useful to obtain a picture of birth and death rates within the population of interest.

## Birth rates

The Director of Public Health within each health authority is notified of all births in the district within 36 hours. The *Public Health Common Data Set* (*PHCDS*) contains local and national statistics on birth rates, abortions, infant mortality rates and maternal ages. These statistics are not recorded at the practice level, but may be a useful starting point if a group of special interest for a health needs assessment was teenage mothers. General fertility rates are measured as the number of births per 1000 women aged 15–44. These rates can be calculated at the practice level over a five-year period, and compared with national and regional figures available from the *PHCDS*.

## Death rates

Information obtained from death certificates is processed nationally by the OPCS. The information is compiled to give district mortality rates which are reported to the Director of Public Health for each health authority. Some practices will have data on both birth and death rates.

   When comparing death rates in different populations it is necessary to adjust crude death rate to take into account the age–sex structure of the populations being compared. Because women have a lower mortality than men, and because mortality increases with age in both sexes, it is necessary to find a way of allowing for differences in the age and sex structure of different populations. For example, many people retire to the coast, so death rates are understandably higher. We allow for this through calculating the standardised mortality ratio (SMR) for the given population. The SMR is defined as:

$$\text{SMR} = \frac{\text{observed number of deaths}}{\text{expected number of deaths}}$$

This figure is usually multiplied by 100 to create whole numbers. The SMR compares the actual death rate with the expected death rate. A standard population would have an SMR of 100, so that an SMR above 100 indicates an excess of actual deaths over expected deaths, while an SMR below 100 indicates fewer actual deaths than would be expected.

**Table 4.1**   Age-standardised mortality rates per 100 000 from different diseases in different geographical areas

|  | England & Wales | Yorkshire RHA | Trent RHA | Grimsby & Scunthorpe |
|---|---|---|---|---|
| Lung cancer | 38.59 | 42.62 | 38.22 | 39.70 |
| Stroke (<65) | 11.89 | 12.63 | 12.81 | 10.67 |
| Breast cancer | 89.68 | 87.73 | 92.45 | 81.84 |
| CHD (<65) | 53.12 | 59.59 | 57.66 | 65.21 |
| Suicide | 11.14 | 11.63 | 10.67 | 7.48 |
| Accidents | 5.65 | 5.71 | 4.80 | 8.06 |

An alternative way of expressing mortality rates is given in the *PHCDS*, which provides age-standardised mortality rates nationally, regionally and locally. An example of the type of information available is shown in Table 4.1. This shows that rates of suicide and stroke in Grimsby and Scunthorpe are lower than the national average, but coronary heart disease is higher, which may be an interesting starting point for health needs assessment in the area.

## Using patient records held within the practice

Sources of data within the practice include the practice computer, community nursing records (Korner returns), audit reports and Prescribing And CosT (PACT) data. Before interpreting data, one must understand the limits of its quality. Until all clinicians are recording all encounters, and all investigations, prescriptions and referrals are reliably entered, analyses of practice data must be viewed with some caution. PACT data is probably one of the most reliable sources of practice data, as most prescriptions are sent to the Prescription Pricing Authority (PPA), the only exception being private prescriptions. Prescribing information is fed back from the PPA to the practice on a three-monthly basis, or as PACT-line data which is sent to the practice every month. Information regarding prescribing may be of use if a health needs assessment is concerned with a group of people with a particular disease, e.g. asthma or diabetes.

Clinical audit data can feed back into health needs assessment and inform the allocation of resources. It is a method used by health professionals to assess, evaluate and improve the care of patients in a systematic way to enhance their health and quality of life. The same guidelines apply for using clinical audit as to all other data generated from within the practice. The audit may focus on a health promotion issue such as smoking. However, in order to use this data to inform decision making, the data should be examined carefully and may need to be validated against manual records.

## Mortality data

Statistics for mortality at a practice level are of limited value because of the small numbers involved. Cause of mortality is not routinely collected by many practices. However, if it is, an increase in mortality is an indicator of morbidity. Of more benefit in health needs assessment are geographical variations of some important diseases (see 'Health and disease data', p. 84).

## Morbidity data

Morbidity is ill health, and in order to know the full extent of ill health it is best to measure morbidity directly, rather than using mortality as a guide to the extent of morbidity. Morbidity ranges in severity from short-term, self-limiting illness (e.g. the common cold) through to chronic conditions that may be long term (e.g. arthritis) to fatal illnesses (e.g. cancer). In order to analyse patterns of morbidity, two concepts are necessary: incidence and prevalence.

*Incidence* is the proportion of the population who are initially free of a condition who develop it over a specified period of time. The numerator of incidence is the number of new cases occurring in the time period, and the denominator is all susceptible people present at the start of the time period (Mulhall 1996).

$$\text{Incidence} = \frac{\text{number of new cases in a fixed time period}}{\text{population at risk}}$$

Incidence rates are useful to planners because they show how many newly diagnosed cases of a disease to expect each year. Changes in incidence rates indicate that a disease is becoming more or less common, or can be a marker of success for health promotion and disease prevention strategies.

If you are planning a screening programme, disease incidence is of immediate interest, for example in determining the cost–benefit of the screening intervention. However, if you are concerned with the provision of services for people who already have a diagnosed health problem, the immediate question is 'How many people have the disease at any point in time?'. You will now be concerned with *prevalence*. Prevalence is the proportion of a defined population who possess a particular condition at a given point in time (point prevalence), or period prevalence refers to the part of the population who possess the condition over a specified period of time.

$$\text{Prevalence} = \frac{\text{number of existing cases}}{\text{total population}}$$

In contrast to incidence, prevalence is determined at a single point in time. Prevalence rates indicate the burden of current disease, disability or handicap. Prevalence rates are particularly useful in identifying health needs of the chronically ill. The Fourth National

General Practice Morbidity Study (MSGP4), conducted by OPCS in 1991, provides comparative rates of incidence and prevalence. Practice rates are not always directly comparable as MSGP4 data were based on consultations, not directly measured morbidity. However, these data are accepted as providing a useful basis for comparison in conjunction with data from other practices. It is possible to standardise the prevalence and incidence figures from a practice to allow for age and sex differences between practices to make more accurate comparisons, although in most cases the crude rates serve well enough.

## Data completeness and accuracy

If the data from general practice computer systems are to be of value in health needs assessment, they must be complete and accurate. Evaluation of the practice database involves a few simple tests, including generating prevalence figures, as in Table 4.2, and comparing them with the national average. If the practice age–sex register is not skewed in any way, then a direct comparison can be made, for example the national average for asthma prevalence is about 10% of the population, and for diabetes mellitus is about 2%. Generally, the chronic disease registers are the most accurate in practices. If the health needs assessment is focusing on a particular 'group of special interest' (see 'Approaches to health needs assessment', p. 75), for example the diabetic patients in the practice, then this data, if accurate, can be very useful.

Lifestyle data is also improving with the advent of new patient clinics, well men and women clinics and elderly checks. These data will provide information about smoking, body mass index, blood pressure, alcohol intake and family history. Family history information should, however, be used with caution as family history status can change over time. For example, if a health needs assessment is focusing on heart disease, then

**Table 4.2**  Prevalence of common diseases diagnosed in general practice

| Diagnosis | Average of four other practices n = 37 455 | Camberwick Green n = 10 552 | Windmill Hill n = 5745 | National figures |
|---|---|---|---|---|
| Asthma | 6.5 | 7.4 | 10.6 | 9.1 |
| Coronary heart disease | 3.0 | 3.2 | 5.7 | 4.3 |
| Dementia | 0.1 | 0.2 | 0.5 | 0.4 |
| Depression | 5.5 | 2.7 | 8.9 | – |
| Diabetes mellitus | 2.1 | 1.8 | 2.6 | 2.7 |
| Glaucoma | 0.5 | 0.8 | 1.4 | 0.3 |
| Hypertension | 5.8 | 6.8 | 8.1 | 10.3 |
| Multiple sclerosis | 0.2 | 0.1 | 0.3 | 0.2 |
| Osteoarthritis (knee) | 1.6 | 2.1 | 2.9 | – |
| Stroke (ever) | 1.1 | 1.3 | 1.5 | 1.3 |
| Stroke in last 2 years | 0.3 | 0.07 | 0.5 | – |

more reliable lifestyle data would be obtained from a questionnaire to patients. Again, if lifestyle data are recorded routinely by all clinicians, they should be checked for accuracy. This can usually be done by running the health promotion audit which is a built-in feature of most GP software systems.

Some diseases, such as diabetes, have a clear link with medication. The recording of diabetes can be checked in a practice by comparing the computer diagnostic register with the repeat prescribing system for all glucosuria and blood glucose diagnostic tests and for all hypoglycaemic agents, including insulin. Where discrepancies are found, the manual records can be checked, and the diagnosis added to the computer records if appropriate. This method can also be used with hypothyroidism and thyroxine prescription, and epilepsy and anti-epileptics (assuming that there is not a valid reason for prescribing an anti-epileptic for any other condition). Auditing these computer-based records will provide an indicator of the general standards of accuracy in the practice information systems.

There are a number of reasons for the prevalence of different disease rates to vary between practices as well as the accuracy and completeness of data. Exercise 1 asks you to explore some figures to identify these reasons.

### Exercise 1

The national figures shown in Table 4.2 are from the Fourth National General Practice Morbidity Study. This table shows the prevalence of ten major diagnoses, using computer diagnostic registers from different practices using the EMIS software system. Prevalence is reported as the percentage of the population with the diagnosis.

Consider the three questions below, bearing in mind all the information available to you from external and internal sources.

1.   Does this table provide useful information in isolation? If not, what further information would be of benefit in analysing the levels of different diagnoses?
2.   The table shows that Windmill Hill has a greater number of people with the diagnosis of asthma compared with national figures, whereas Camberwick Green is lower. What further information would be useful in considering the reasons why, and what are the implications for diagnosis and recording?
3.   There are no national figures for depression. Can you suggest why, and consider the reasons for, the large inter-practice variation in the prevalence for depression?

## Methods for collecting primary data

The approaches to data collection described in the previous section are very good ways of identifying major issues and measuring the size of the problem. However, there are times when we need to know more about the background or about the impact of these problems. As we have seen, public and practice records can tell us about the main health problems and the numbers of people suffering from these problems. However, they do not tell us about the impact of these problems on the lives of individuals. When more detailed information of this type is required, consideration should be given to using first-hand methods of data collection. In this section we will consider four approaches to data collection which can be used in health needs assessment:

(1)   direct observation
(2)   surveys
(3)   individual interviews
(4)   focus groups.

In this section we briefly consider the use of different approaches to the collection of primary (empirical) data. Further guidance on these methods is available elsewhere in this series.

## Direct observation

Not all methods of primary data collection require contact with human beings. Observation of the environment can provide valuable background information about the area where a health needs assessment is taking place. Observation can also serve as a technique for verifying or questioning information provided in face-to-face encounters.

Direct observation can include broad descriptions of the key features of the area. For example, whether the area is inner city, urban or rural; the geographical location; the size of the population. It can describe the key components of the area: the main industries; type of housing. The availability of services can be identified: number, type and location of healthcare facilities such as hospitals and health centres; leisure facilities; shopping centres. Observations can also be more detailed, focusing on the physical features of a locality and their relevance to a particular health issue. For example, if the focus was on accident prevention among children, observations would include roads, gardens and public playing areas. Box 4.7 lists some of the features on which observation data might be collected as part of a health needs assessment.

It may be possible to include photographs or even to use video technology when using observational data to illustrate a community profile. It is also possible to directly observe the work of primary care practitioners as they interact with their clients.

### Exercise 2

Box 4.7 lists some of the features that might be observed and included in a health needs assessment. Make your own copy of the box with the contents of the right-hand column deleted. Think about the area where you live and make notes about the key features using the categories listed in the left-hand column.

---

**Box 4.7**    Features for inclusion in observational data

| Observation category | Examples of information for inclusion |
| --- | --- |
| General appearance | City, urban or rural<br>Size |
| Population | Factors likely to affect make-up of population, e.g. elderly person's housing (older people); university (young people) |
| Leisure | Leisure centres, entertainment facilities |
| Health services | Location of nearest hospital(s)<br>Number and location of general practices<br>Facilities provided by health centres |
| Housing | Ratio of owner occupiers to tenants<br>Types of housing |
| Income levels | Types of employment<br>House prices<br>Types of shops |
| Communications | Transport facilities<br>Major roads |
| Retail outlets | Types of shops and price range<br>Food outlets (e.g. fast food) |
| Work related | Major industries<br>Facilities for the unemployed |

---

## Surveys

In health needs assessment, much information can be gained through analysing routinely available statistics and observing the neighbourhood. However, you may also need to ask some direct questions of the people you are concerned about. Perhaps you want to know what social support is available to carers in your neighbourhood, for example, or how many older people cannot shop for themselves. You may wish to identify gaps in the services your health centre provides, or to find out how many people are interested in getting fit or eating more healthily.

The survey is a method of gathering information which will immediately spring to mind. We are all familiar with this technique, having no doubt been stopped on the high street and asked to give our opinion on everything from new flavour chocolate bars to the state of the economy. If we have used the health service ourselves in recent years, we may well have filled in a questionnaire to let the service providers know what we think of them. A survey can be defined very simply as the collection of information in a standardised form from groups of people. Typically, the researcher surveys a selection of individuals from a known population and collects a relatively small range of data (Robson 1993). The survey method is usually based on a questionnaire that can be completed by the respondents themselves, or in a structured interview conducted by the researcher or their assistants. The four main methods of collecting survey data are:

(1)   face-to-face interviews
(2)   telephone interviews
(3)   postal surveys
(4)   self-completion questionnaires.

Surveys can be carried out for *descriptive* purposes. The decennial census is a good example of a descriptive survey. It asks a range of questions about households and the individuals within them which can then be used to describe the population. In health needs assessment, you may wish to carry out a survey which asks people to tell you about their housing or employment situations; you will then be able to use this information to profile your target population in greater depth than routinely collected information allows.

You may also carry out a survey to explore the *consumer view*. You may wish to find out about peoples' views of the services at your health centre, or ask them to express their own understanding of their health needs.

Surveys can be also be used to *analyse* the relationship between 'variables', or different elements of the information you have collected. At this point, survey design gets more complicated and requires some understanding of the statistical techniques used for data analysis.

Before you embark on a survey, it is essential that you reflect on what exactly it is you are hoping to achieve. Exercise 3, which follows, will help you to do this by asking you to work through a number of relevant questions. The advantages of survey research are that studies can be designed to cover large numbers of people; it is possible to generalise to the larger population through appropriate sampling; and standardised data can be easier and quicker to analyse. However, in assessing health need we must always remember that people might be influenced by how they are feeling at that moment, or immediate problems among their family and friends. Also, respondents may have difficulty in evaluating their needs if they have no knowledge of how services could be provided differently.

The discussion above is limited, and it is suggested that you obtain advice before embarking on a survey which will be very demanding of time and money.


## Individual interviews

Interviews can be highly structured, semi-structured or unstructured. *Structured interviews* consist of the interviewer asking each respondent the same questions in the same way. A tightly structured schedule of questions is used very much like a questionnaire. The questions may even be phrased in such a way that a limited range of responses can be elicited; for example, 'Do you think that health services in this area are excellent, good, average or poor?'. Bearing in mind the cost of conducting a series of one-to-one interviews, the researcher planning to use structured interviews should consider carefully whether the information could be more efficiently collected using questionnaires.

*Semi-structured interviews* (sometimes referred to as focused interviews) involve a series of open-ended questions based on the topic areas the researcher wants to cover. The open-ended nature of the question defines the topic under investigation but provides opportunities for both interviewer and interviewee to discuss some topics in more detail. If the interviewee has difficulty answering a question or provides only a brief response, the interviewer can use cues or prompts to encourage the interviewee to consider the question further.

*Unstructured interviews* (sometimes referred to as 'depth' or 'in-depth' interviews) have very little structure at all. The interviewer goes into the interview with the aim of discussing a limited number of topics, as few as one or two, and frames the questions on the basis of the interviewee's previous response. Although only one or two topics are discussed, they are covered in great detail. The interview might begin with the interviewer saying 'I'd like to hear your views on the health needs of people in this area'. Subsequent questions would depend on how the interviewee responded.

Semi-structured interviews tend to work well in health needs assessments as the interviewer can decide in advance what areas to cover but is open and receptive to unexpected information from the interviewee.

An example of an interview schedule is shown in Box 4.8. This was used in a general practice-based health needs assessment carried out in Grimsby.

---

**Box 4.8**    Example of an interview schedule

| *Main questions* | *Prompts* |
|---|---|
| Do you think the people in Grimsby are healthy? | |
| What do you think are the main health problems in this area? | Individual age groups, lifestyle, special needs groups, worst problems/highest priority |
| What are the main social problems in Grimsby? | Unemployment, single parent/teenage pregnancy, poverty, drug/alcohol abuse, housing |
| Do you think the health and social services are meeting the needs of the local community? | Different services, hospital, GP, social services, community services, allocation of resources, accessibility, acceptability |
| Do you think there are enough community facilities to keep people healthy? | Health facilities, community clinics and screening, social/leisure facilities, accessibility |
| If you had a magic wand, could you suggest one change you would like to make to the health service? | |

Semi-structured interviews should not be seen as a soft option requiring little forethought. Good-quality qualitative interviews are the result of rigorous preparation. The development of the interview schedule, conducting the interview and analysing the interview data all require careful consideration and preparation.

## Focus groups

Sometimes it is preferable to collect information from groups of people rather than from a series of individuals. Focus groups represent a method of data collection which has been widely used in the private sector over the past few decades, particularly in market research. Focus groups are increasingly used in the public sector to obtain the 'user voice' in the evaluation and planning of services.

Focus groups have a great deal of potential in the process of health needs assessment. They can be held at an early, exploratory stage when initial clues and insights are needed or when there is a lack of communication between people which could be overcome by facilitating discussion. For example, the views of both parents and teachers on the health needs of young people could be explored in a focus group. Part of the discussion might include the expectations that each group has of each other in terms of the type of information they expect young people to be provided with. Focus groups can be particularly useful when the research team wants to collect ideas about the type of services which should be provided after identifying health needs. For example, after identifying a need for a mobile well woman or well man clinic in rural areas, a focus group could explore what sort of services should be provided or which geographical areas are in most need. Kreuger (1994) provides an excellent practical guide to using focus groups.

## Combining data collection methods

Health needs assessment is best carried out using a combination of methods. Often, quantitative and qualitative data complement each other by providing insights into the size and nature of health needs. Comprehensive health needs assessment which promotes community participation and development can be very demanding in terms of time and commitment. Rapid appraisal is a technique which has been developed to obtain information about a set of problems in a short period and without a large expenditure of professional time and finance (Ong 1996).

Rapid appraisal is the first step in the process of planning health interventions for specific communities. Information is collected from existing records and from mapping the social and environmental characteristics of the area. However, the techniques used in rapid appraisal also access the 'user voice' and explore the community's own perceptions of need and priorities. The strength of feeling among local residents is assessed through semi-structured interviews with the following 'key informants':

- professionals working in the community such as teachers, police officers and health visitors
- elected and self-elected leaders such as the local MP, councillors and leaders of tenants' associations
- people who are important within informal networks and who play a central role in local communications such as shopkeepers, hairdressers and publicans.

Rapid appraisal is carried out by a team of researchers, whose members may include primary healthcare professionals, representatives of health authorities and representatives of local authorities from a wide range of departments. As well as being a relatively quick and focused approach to health needs assessment, rapid appraisal also reflects the primary healthcare principles of equity, community participation and multisectoral cooperation. However, it is worth bearing in mind that this approach can identify conflicts within the neighbourhood as well as key priorities. For example, primary healthcare practitioners may wish to expand the service they offer to homeless people, whereas local residents may want to see fewer 'rough sleepers' using local hostels. Despite this warning, the techniques used to carry out a rapid appraisal do allow unmet needs and local priorities to be identified. The data obtained can be used to construct an information pyramid, which will be discussed in the next section of this chapter.

# Summary

Health needs assessment can be carried out using a variety of methods. It is important that the method(s) selected are appropriate to the type of information required, the population being assessed and the resources of the research team. Exercise 3 provides an opportunity to consolidate your understanding of the advantages and disadvantages of the different methods.

## *Exercise 3*

Look at the proposed health needs assessment projects listed below. In each case consider the kind of information required, appropriate methods for collecting data and the resource implications of the selected approach. You may consider your response from a practice, locality or district perspective.

Project 1: an assessment of the needs of teenage mothers.
Project 2: plans to develop health promotion services for men.
Project 3: a comprehensive health check system for over 75s.

# Putting health needs assessment into practice

This section explores the interpretation of data collected in health needs assessments and considers how the findings can be used to plan services.

## Interpretation of data

Before interpreting data collected in a health needs assessment, one must understand the limits of its quality. For example, practice data (as described in 'Using public health data and patient records', p. 80) must be properly validated before being relied on – the quality of data retrieved reflects the quality of data entry. It might be supposed that external data, such as census data, are much more accurate. However, no survey has a complete response rate, especially questionnaires. The census is more complete than most, but it has a low response in inner cities and among ethnic minorities. All data sources have limitations, which become more obvious as the scientific accuracy with which data are analysed increases. Nevertheless, health needs assessment deals in rounder, larger verities which recognise limitations while making the best of all information available.

*Triangulation* can be used to both analyse and present results. Triangulation refers to the use of a combination of approaches to explore one set of research questions, as is often appropriate in health needs assessment. Triangulation can refer to a combination of different methods, or to the different data sources used to explore the same phenomenon. It is a process for judging the validity of the different methods and sources by comparing them (Mason 1996).

Given the speculative nature of much of the data used in health needs assessment, 'fact' is hard to establish from a single source. Whenever possible, more than one data source should be explored to substantiate a conclusion. In some instances, such robustness is not possible, but one reason for adopting a range of methodologies and tapping a number of sources is to increase the reliability and validity of data. Some examples of triangulation of data are listed in Table 4.3.

### The concept of an information pyramid

The various forms of information collected in a health needs assessment can be brought together to form an information pyramid (Figure 4.1). This concept has its origin in rapid appraisal (Annett and Rifkin 1988) but the principle can be applied to health needs assessment where other methods have been used. The pyramid shape reminds health managers that success depends on a planning process which rests on a strong community information base, and that the amount of information needed about each area is relative to its position in the pyramid. It is the quality of the information, not the quantity, that is most crucial.

**Table 4.3**   Triangulation in health needs assessment

|                | Practice data | External statistics | Rapid appraisal |
|----------------|---------------|---------------------|-----------------|
| Deprivation    |               | 60% of population are social classes 3M, 4 & 5, compared with national average of 46%. Jarman and Townsend indices show the practice covers wards that are more deprived than the general area, and the average for England and Wales | High unemployment, teenage pregnancies and single-parent families |
| Lifestyle      | 40% of men & 35% of women smoke | National and local average of 30% | Poor diet, lack of exercise, high alcohol intake and high levels of smoking and drug abuse |
| Morbidity      | No practice data to support this as numbers would be too low to draw useful conclusions | Coronary heart disease age-standardised mortality rate is 65 per 100 000 per year compared with a national level of 53 | Coronary heart disease, respiratory problems and mental health problems |
| Workload       | High list size per doctor (approx 2500) | National average list size of 1800 | |
| Chronic disease management | 80% of patients with hypertension –72% with hypertension had been reviewed within the last year | | Generally interviewees were complimentary about primary care services and acknowledged that patients received high-quality care |

The foundation of the pyramid is built on information about community composition, organisation and capacity to act. As the planning process is based on community involvement and contribution to a plan of action for health improvements, it is necessary for health workers to know about the community in which they are working, including the strengths and weaknesses of the community leadership, organisations and structures.

The next level describes the socio-ecological factors which influence health, including the physical environment, socio-economic conditions and disease and disability. Information at this level is required in order to investigate the potentials and barriers which exist for community improvements. Data on the physical environment seek to identify any environmental causes of disease and disability, for example problems such as overcrowding and pollution. Data on the social aspects focus on traditional beliefs and values which facilitate or impede behavioural changes. An analysis of economic aspects highlights

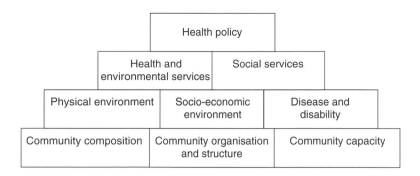

**Figure 4.1** Information pyramid

income sources, earning potential and the economic opportunities of various community groups.

The third level concerns data on the existence, coverage, accessibility and acceptability of services. These include health services, environmental services and social services such as education and assistance for the disabled. The final level at which some general knowledge is required is that concerning national, regional and local policies about health improvements. Information on these policies will provide background on the 'political' commitment to primary healthcare. Making a case that the findings of the health needs assessment are directly related to problems and priorities recognised at policy-making levels will increase the likelihood that resources will be allocated or diverted.

## Using the results in practice

Once the data for health needs assessment have been collected and analysed it is possible to seek solutions to the identified problems. Many ways of identifying priorities involve a form of ranking. They include prioritising based on the size of the health problem (prevalence and incidence), its severity in terms of morbidity or mortality, the availability of effective interventions, the feasibility of the work entailed for the primary healthcare team, the level of group interest and the costs and resources required (Gillam and Murray 1996). The prioritising process should include as many of the primary healthcare team as possible, in order to take account of current workload and set realistic targets. Audit and evaluation are an integral part of the planning cycle – they answer the question of 'whether you have got where you want to go' – and should be specifically focused on the priority needs identified, rather than personal interest or choice.

During the process of health needs assessment, team members will probably have developed ideas about how to tackle the problems identified. When the team reaches this stage they must decide what interventions they are prepared to undertake. Annett and Rifkin (1988) suggest that information collected by rapid appraisal techniques provides a wide variety of data which can be used to develop a feasibility matrix which enables planners to decide the priority on which to place suggestions for future actions. Each intervention can be examined for the following characteristics:

| | |
|---|---|
| *Health benefit* | What is the overall health impact? |
| *Community capacity* | How committed is the community to solving the problems and what can they contribute to the solutions? |
| *Sustainability* | Can the intervention be maintained and at what cost? |
| *Equity* | Which income groups are likely to benefit most? |
| *Cost* | What are the initial capital and manpower costs? |
| *Time for benefit* | How long will it be before changes are noticeable? |

Each intervention is scored as '+' for low, '++' for medium and '+++' for high. The highest total score is given the highest priority.

Table 4.4 provides an example of how a priority matrix was used to consider whether or not to set up a community-based women's health group following a locality-based health needs assessment. As the table shows, the proposed intervention scored a maximum +++ in four out of six categories and ++ in the remaining two. The women's health group appears to be highly feasible. Whether or not it would be identified as a priority would depend on how it compares with other proposals.

**Table 4.4**  A priority matrix assessing the feasibility of a women's health group

| Characteristics | Relevant considerations | Score |
|---|---|---|
| Health benefit | The group can address a wide range of health issues concerning women and their families. | +++ |
| Community capacity | Many women have said they would like a group but they might not feel able, or wish to make, lifestyle changes. | ++ |
| Sustainability | Two health promotion specialists employed to deal with women's health are currently half way through two-year contracts so staff are available for at least the next year. Premises not a problem – local community centre. Maintaining a membership might be a problem. | ++ |
| Equity | All income groups have expressed a need. Lower social groups resident in locality can easily access community centre. Crèche facilities could be made available. | +++ |
| Cost | Minimal start-up costs. Health promotion specialists already employed and experienced at group work in other localities. | +++ |
| Time for benefit | Take up of breast screening and cervical screening immediately quantifiable. Other outcome measures would need to be developed. | +++ |

## The role of the primary healthcare team

It has already been stated that health needs assessment should be carried out by teams to ensure commitment to the principles behind the process. Using the findings to plan services should also be a team activity. The information collected may suggest the need for changes in the way services are organised and delivered. This may include suggestions about who provides a particular service. For example, it may be that work undertaken by GPs could be undertaken by practice nurses or that clinical staff are involved in clerical tasks which would be more cost-effectively performed by administrative staff. Sharing the results of the health needs assessment among the team and discussing as a team possible ways of responding will help everyone to understand why change may be necessary and of mutual benefit. One way to get the whole team involved is to organise an 'Away Day' where group facilitators enable all team members to consider the results of the health needs assessment, identify priorities and start to plan.

## Conclusion

Primary healthcare professionals would not wish to undertake a health needs assessment unless there were clear benefits to be achieved. Decisions must be taken which affect the range and quality of primary care services which their patients receive. The information pyramid can help community health professionals to focus on the 'what, why and how' of health needs assessment in primary care.

Primary care is facing an agenda for change which is both exciting and alarming. Practitioners need, more than ever, to understand the principles of clinical and cost-effectiveness, efficiency and equity in healthcare provision. Primary care is being asked to lead the National Health Service into the next century. Needs assessment is the cornerstone of primary care-led purchasing and commissioning, and the key to service provision which is sensitive to local conditions. A successful health needs assessment will utilise the appropriate methods to collect the appropriate data, and will follow through with a genuine commitment to improving public health.

# Answers to exercises

The exercises for this chapter are to a large extent based on self-selected examples. It is not feasible, therefore, to provide specific answers to all questions. You should, however, draw on the guidelines provided in the text when approaching them. The following comments can be made for Exercises 1 and 3.

## Exercise 1

1.  Age–sex register for all practices:
    -   are there any age groups under- or over-represented?
2.  Age–sex register of practice populations:
    -   do all clinicians record all diagnoses in a standard, retrievable way?

   – is there an asthma clinic, with a specialist asthma nurse, at any of the practices?
   – are patients encouraged to attend clinics, and are rates of diagnosis therefore increased?
   – does Camberwick Green have a protocol for asthma?

3. Depression diagnosis has a certain stigma which GPs may be reluctant to attach, therefore figures are low and depression is under-represented. As practices may not record on the computer all cases of depression, it is difficult for studies such as the Fourth National General Practice Morbidity Study to collect and compare data accurately. There are many different Read codes for depression, and diagnosis is subjective. Inter-practice variation can be accounted for by all these factors.

## Exercise 3

Project 1:
- demographic or practice data on the number of teenage mothers locally
- deprivation scores in the areas where they live
- focus groups with teenage mothers
- focus groups or individual interviews with people who come into contact with young mothers.

Project 2:
- epidemiological data about the main health problems affecting this group compared with local or national averages
- individual interviews to consider health promotion approaches
- survey of men registered in the practice(s) to assess potential uptake.

Project 3:
- epidemiological data about the main health problems affecting this group compared with local or national averages
- postal survey or face-to-face interviews as part of current health check to assess unmet need.

# References

Annett H and Rifkin S (1988) *Improving Urban Health – Guidelines for Rapid Appraisal to Assess Community Health Needs*. World Health Organization, Geneva.

Burton P (1993) *Community Profiling: A Guide to Identifying Local Needs*. School for Advanced Urban Studies, University of Bristol, Bristol.

Department of Health (1992) *The Health of the Nation: A Strategy for Health in England*. HMSO, London.

Department of Health (1996) *Primary Care: Delivering the Future*. HMSO, London.

Doyal L and Gough I (1991) *A Theory of Human Need*. Macmillan, London.

Gillam S J and Murray S A (1996) *Needs Assessment in General Practice*. Occasional Paper 73. Royal College of General Practitioners, London.

Hawe P, Dageling D and Hall J (1990) *Evaluating Health Promotion: A Health Worker's Guide*. MacLennan and Petty, Sydney.

Hawtin M, Hughes G and Percy-Smith J (1994) *Community Profiling: Auditing Social Needs*. Open University Press, Buckingham.

Kreuger R A (1994) *Focus Groups: A Practical Guide for Applied Research* (2nd edn). Sage Publications, London.

Lightfoot J (1995) Identifying needs and setting priorities: issues of theory, policy and practice. *Health and Social Care in the Community.* **3**: 105–14.

Mason J (1996) *Qualitative Researching*. Sage Publications, London.

Muir B (1996) *Developing a Health Profile for General Practice*. Unpublished thesis, Nottingham School of Public Health, University of Nottingham, Nottingham.

Mulhall A (1996) *Epidemiology, Nursing and Healthcare: A New Perspective*. Macmillan Press, Basingstoke.

NHSME (1993) *New World, New Opportunities: Nursing in Primary Health*. Department of Health, London.

Nicholas A (1996) Making it happen: community nurses' public health role. *Health Visitor.* **69**(1): 28–30.

Ong B N (1996) *Rapid Appraisal and Health Policy*. Chapman and Hall, London.

Payne J N, Coy J, Patterson S and Milner P C (1994) Is use of hospital services a proxy for morbidity? A small area comparison of the prevalence of arthritis, depression, dyspepsia, obesity and respiratory disease with in-patient admission rates for these disorders in England. *Journal of Epidemiology and Community Health.* **48**: 74–8.

Peckham S and Macdonald J (1996) *Primary Care and Public Health*. Report to Public Health Trust Steering Group. Public Health Alliance, Birmingham.

Percy-Smith J and Sanderson I (1992) *Understanding Local Needs*. Institute for Public Policy Research, London.

Pickin C and St Leger S (1993) *Assessing Health Need Using the Life-cycle Framework*. Open University Press, Buckingham.

Robinson J and Elkan R (1996) *Health Needs Assessment: Theory and Practice*. Churchill Livingstone, London.

Robson C (1993) *Real World Research*. Blackwell, Oxford.

Ross F and Mackenzie A (1996) *Nursing in Primary Health Care: Policy into Practice*. Routledge, London.

Sheffield Health Authority (1996) *A 'Toolkit' for Health Needs Assessment in Primary Care*. Sheffield Health, LAPIS, Sheffield.

Streiner D L and Norman G R (1996) *PDQ Epidemiology* (2nd edn). Mosby, London.

Unwin N, Carr S, Leeson J and Pless-Mulloli T (1997) *An Introductory Study Guide to Public Health and Epidemiology*. Open University Press, Buckingham.

# Further reading and resources

Annett H and Rifkin S (1988) *Improving Urban Health – Guidelines for Rapid Appraisal to Assess Community Health Needs*. World Health Organization, Geneva.

Gillam S J and Murray S A (1996) *Needs Assessment in General Practice*. Occasional Paper 73. Royal College of General Practitioners, London.

Kreuger R A (1994) *Focus Groups: A Practical Guide for Applied Research* (2nd edn). Sage Publications, London.

Mays N and Pope C (eds) (1996) *Qualitative Research in Health Care*. BMJ Publishing Group, London.

Murray S A, Tapson J, Turnbull L *et al.* (1994) Listening to local voices: adapting rapid appraisal to assess health and social needs in general practice. *British Medical Journal*. **308**: 698–700.

Murray S A and Graham L J C (1995) Practice-based health needs assessment: use of four methods in a small neighbourhood. *British Medical Journal*. **310**: 1443–8.

NHSME (1992) *Local Voices. The Views of Local People in Purchasing for Health*. Department of Health, London.

Pickin C and St Leger S (1993) *Assessing Health Need Using the Life-cycle Framework*. Open University Press, Buckingham.

Pringle M, Ward P and Chivers C (1995) Assessment of the completeness and accuracy of computer medical records in four practices committed to recording data on computer. *British Journal of General Practice*. **45**: 537–41.

Robinson J and Elkan R (1996) *Health Needs Assessment: Theory and Practice*. Churchill Livingstone, London.

## Health needs assessment studies

You should be able to find information about health needs assessments undertaken locally by contacting your health authority, local authority, NHS community trust and university departments of general practice, primary care or public health. Examples of information available include:

Pringle M, Hammersley V, Brown K and Carmichael C (1997) *Health Needs in Primary Care*. Unpublished report. University of Nottingham, Nottingham.

Community Profile Steering Group (1996) *Community Profile – The Sherwood Estate*. Nottingham City Council, Nottingham.

## Health authorities

Every health authority holds information on local, regional and national morbidity and mortality figures. This information can be found in documents such as the *Public Health Common Data Set* and the *Fourth National Morbidity Study*.

Some health authorities may prepare additional information based on locality profiles. For example, Nottingham Health Authority have produced *Health Maps of Nottingham* which analyses census data, deprivation rates, morbidity and mortality rates by electoral ward.

## Local authorities

Local authorities hold census data and they may have analysed the data contained within the census at electoral ward level.

# CHAPTER FIVE

# Presenting and disseminating research

*Jane Schober and Andy Farrington*

## Introduction

It is commonly recognised that research and research projects are now activities undertaken by more and more healthcare professionals in primary care and other fields. Whilst this is clearly crucial to the underpinning of evidence-based research practice, the results of such labours need to be written up clearly for others to see, understand and apply to practice, as well as disseminating the findings and outcomes of such research as widely as possible.

The general purpose of a research project is to gather information about an issue or problem and construct a report or article to disseminate the outcomes of the appropriate research process. In addition, it must be remembered that any research activity has personal and organisational benefits. These are summarised in Box 5.1 and you will see that they contain common features that illustrate components, which strengthen any research culture.

This chapter is for practitioners working in primary healthcare settings. It will help in writing up a research project and includes some tips on seeking publication of the final report. It will also give you the opportunity to study and understand the features of a research project which consists of several parts:

- how a research project can contribute to professional practice
- the opportunities available to undertake and execute a research project
- guidelines for writing up a research project which will ensure continuity of presentation, coherence and flow of material
- disseminating research outcomes, including local and national strategies.

---

**Box 5.1**   Benefits of research

| *Personal* | *Organisational* |
|---|---|

*Personal*
- Improving patient care
- Initiating change
- Finding out
- The search for meaning
- The need to understand
- Looking for causal relationships
- Testing theories
- Discovering the new
- Self-esteem and kudos
- As part of a course of study
- Specialist area of interest

*Organisational*
- Improving healthcare and well-being
- Planning for change and innovation
- Informing policy and practice
- Knowledge-based approach
- Encouraging an evaluative culture
- Responding to policies and demands
- Reacting to public opinion
- Delivering measurable results
- Quality and audit
- Cost-effectiveness
- Developing evidence-based practice

---

# Writing up a research project

Although there is a range of approaches to research, when it comes to communicating the details of research activities through the written word there are a number of pointers you should consider. It has long been a criticism of researchers that they do not communicate their research clearly and in a user-friendly manner.

With this in mind, this section will provide you with guidelines that will help you both to understand the research project or reports you encounter as part of your professional reading and to organise, structure and communicate your own reports in an appropriate manner.

There are several ways of communicating the outcomes of a research exercise in writing. The most common is the research report, others include the research dissertation, research abstracts, research summaries and research articles. Although they have certain features in common, there are also clear differences which are outlined here.

## The research report

A research report is a highly structured piece of writing that clearly states the purpose, findings and outcomes of research activity. A report may be written for a range of reasons and for a variety of audiences, therefore its length, style and detail may vary greatly. Research reports are usually produced for such groups as service users, multidisciplinary colleagues and fellow professionals and as a result of commissioned research.

The report is shaped and influenced by:

- the questions that need a response or answer
- the target audience

- the background to its production, for example any related research, theoretical perspectives and how the research was organised and managed
- the style needed to communicate findings in a way that will maximise their understanding.

A report inevitably summarises key aspects of the research process undertaken to complete it. This is particularly so if a report is needed at, for example, a committee meeting, a seminar or a conference where time, attention spans and other agendas may affect the detail presented. Where a report is used as a summary and reference document, the researcher often has the opportunity to describe, discuss, elaborate and evaluate aspects of the research in relation to the audience.

It is important in these circumstances that a full and detailed report has been prepared first, from which the summary is extracted. This ensures that the audience is able to access the details to explain the context, scope, significance and implications of the findings. The main features of a report will depend on its themes and purpose. Marshall and Rowland (1993) suggest the following structure:

(1)   the title
(2)   abstract
(3)   the research problem or question
(4)   background and reasons for the study
(5)   methodology
(6)   results
(7)   analysis of the findings
(8)   discussion
(9)   conclusions
(10)   recommendations.

These subheadings are explained fully in 'Contents of a written report', p. 109.

Within a report, much emphasis is placed on the outcomes and results. It is these that the commissioner of the report is waiting for. However, the credibility of the results will depend on how all other aspects of the work have been planned, managed, executed and resourced. Reports are usually shorter than dissertations and the form and style of a report may be less formal and academic to meet the needs and interests of the audience. Accessibility is all-important and conciseness and preciseness along with clear visual representation of findings are essential characteristics.
Key bullet point summaries of:

- findings
- implications
- recommendations

for example, can alert the audience to significant features which can be followed up in the main report as well as being tools for focused discussion.

## The research dissertation

There are marked parallels between a research report and a dissertation. This is particularly so in relation to its structure and organisation. Dissertations are a common feature of undergraduate and postgraduate degree studies. Whether undertaking a first degree or a higher degree, the management of a research dissertation bears similar characteristics.

Where research reports and dissertations tend to differ is in their length and complexity. As dissertations are produced as part of an academic exercise, there is a need to explain, qualify and justify aspects of the study, for instance the methodology. These may be reduced and sometimes omitted from a report.

Empirical studies are usually based on factual information, experience or observation. Part of the process is to gather information and data about a problem, to question or to update previous research. Empirical studies incorporate a range of research methodologies, including surveys, case studies, ethnography and experimental designs which may influence the form of presentation of the dissertation.

It is not uncommon for undergraduate students to undertake a dissertation by literature review. This approach facilitates detailed analysis of the literature pertaining to aspects of practice, treatments, historical perspectives and theory. Analysis of theory, previous research, experiences and incidents, amongst other things, gives students the opportunity to develop academic skills relating to the in-depth study of a topic. A common format for the literature review is as follows:

(1)    literature searching and review
(2)    critical analysis of previous research
(3)    concept analysis and theoretical understanding
(4)    comparative analysis of previous work
(5)    discussing the significance of previous findings
(6)    identifying areas for future study.

The extent of the literature search is central to the quality of the review and is often more extensive than a search and analysis undertaken for an empirical study.

The action approach to research is mainly concerned with the evaluation of practice by the practising professional. Action research has its origins in the teaching profession and has gained popularity among healthcare professionals as a means of studying their own practice.

## Common features of research reports and dissertations

Any research which is formally presented needs to adopt key attributes to ensure clarity, credibility and accessibility. Edwards and Talbot (1994) suggest the following common features:

• readability – so that it can be clearly and quickly understood

- clear organisation – so that the reader is easily led through the text
- a logical reference system – so that the reader can quickly follow up any references
- information presented in a logical order – so that the reader does not at any point have to guess, for example, how the data was analysed or the conclusion was reached
- substantiation – so that each claim can be seen to be based on evidence.

It is not uncommon for reports to emerge following the completion of a dissertation. This is a very useful tool for disseminating the process and outcomes of the research, for presentation to peers, colleagues in the organisation where the research took place and as a part of the preparation process for possible publication or conference presentation.

## Exercise 1

Reports and dissertations relating to primary healthcare would usually contribute to the expanding body of knowledge about healthcare in community settings. When writing up a report or dissertation relating to primary healthcare, what key themes and perspectives could be usefully addressed to emphasise current professional issues?

# Contents of a written report

This section provides guidelines on presenting a detailed, written research report. You will have seen in the previous section that there are marked similarities between a research report and a research dissertation. Indeed, some sources appear to use the terms interchangeably. This section covers both and will highlight those areas that need elaboration for a dissertation. It is worth noting that many computer software packages now provide template guides and interactive support to format reports and/or dissertations.

Presentation is important but not as important as:

- content
- clarity
- order of argument.

Not all reports and dissertations take the same form and it is difficult to cover all possibilities. **You should therefore use your discretion in following this guide and, if you have any doubts, seek advice from your supervisor and always check through any guidelines you have been given.**

## Layout

The following is the usual order of the elements in a research report but will vary depending on method, as in the case of a literature review or experiment for instance.

## Title page

This should have a balanced appearance and consist of:

*   the title which should be descriptive yet reasonably concise
*   the full name of the author and qualifications if necessary
*   the organisation for which the research is undertaken
*   the month and year of submission.

## Contents table

This should list the chapters and their main subdivisions as well as the page number on which each begins. In addition, chapter headings should be short, descriptive and to the point, items such as acknowledgements and appendices should be listed and all pages must be numbered. Illustrations, tables and figures must be clearly labelled and related to the text.

It is common practice to assign Arabic numbers (1,2,3, etc.) to chapters and lower-case Roman numerals (i, ii, iii, etc.) or small letters (a,b,c, etc.) to subdivisions or separate points. An alternative method is to number sections as subsets of chapters, as for example:

*   1.1, 1.2, 1.2.1 in Chapter 1
*   2.1, 2.2, 2.2.1 in Chapter 2

and so on, using a decimal notation.

## List of tables and figures

It is helpful both for the author and readers if table and figure numbers relate as closely as possible to the relevant part of the text, thus, the first table in Chapter 3 might be numbered 3.1.

## Acknowledgements

It is courteous to mention anyone who has provided significant help, facilities and resources for the research. Sponsors will expect to receive recognition for their support.

## Abstract (essential for dissertations)

This is a summary of about 500 words, indicating the main points and conclusions in the order described in the report. It should also mention techniques and equipment used, and be in complete sentences, not in note form. Edwards and Talbot (1994) suggest information about each of the following should be included:

*   the research question
*   the theoretical framework

- the design of the study, including sample size and methodology
- main findings and their implications.

## Abbreviations

Any abbreviations used should be explained where they are first used, for example Department of Health (DoH). If they are repeated throughout the text it is useful to provide a list at the beginning of the work.

## Main text

Guidelines for research projects follow, which are particularly relevant to dissertations and detailed research reports. Each of the following subheadings may be listed as chapters, *particularly in dissertations*. Although there cannot be any rigid rules for the layout of the main text, the following points may be helpful.

*Introduction:*
- background to the problem/area of study, including a brief statement of what is being investigated
- the rationale for the study – reasons for undertaking the work
- statements concerning the significance of the study and the purposes of conducting it
- if you are using a formal theory, theoretical framework or a conceptual framework, this should be explained (*essential for dissertations*)
- definitions of concepts and terms with appropriate discussion to set them in the context of your research (*essential for dissertations*)
- hypothesis (not relevant to all research studies)
- the aims of the project.

*Literature review*
This section should be comprehensive and relevant, and include summaries of other related studies, articles and texts related to the area of research. Deficiencies or gaps in the literature should be highlighted so that the need for this particular study can be demonstrated. Students undertaking a *dissertation by literature review* will also need to address, in detail, the following:

- the structure and organisation of the review
- the comprehensiveness of the review
- the analysis of the literature.

*Study design/methodology*
This chapter should be organised in a way that suits the particular study. *Theoretical justification for the method used would normally be given in a dissertation.* In terms of the study design/methodology, the following points need to be considered:

- a detailed description and justification of the data collection methods used (for example, questionnaire, measuring tools or interviews)

- the sampling approach explained and discussed
- a description of the pilot study (if undertaken), and an explanation of whether it did or did not lead to changes in the main study (but not including data from the pilot study)
- issues relating to validity, sensitivity and reliability
- a detailed description and justification of the data analysis methods used (for example, statistical tools, content analysis or constant comparative methods to find categories and themes)
- ethical issues, including how ethical approval was sought and details of confirmation (as necessary)
- specific limitations which become apparent may be discussed here or in the final section.

The introduction and literature review inform the development of the study, particularly the aims, objectives, hypothesis and methodology.

*Data collection*
This section should contain sufficient information to convince your reader that your data collection methods support the research approach taken. There should also be sufficient detail to allow for replication of the study. In this respect it should include, as appropriate, details of:

- access to the site
- permission to collect data
- access to respondents/subjects/clients/patients
- the where, when and (if appropriate) time of data collection
- sensitivity to the needs, rights, privacy and anonymity of the respondents
- ethical issues arising out of any of these points.

*Findings/results*
The presentation of the findings of a research project is essential to the clear communication of the outcomes of the data collection process. A combination of visual and literary description will ensure that the information presented is unambiguous and that all outcomes are included.

The presentation should be:

- factual
- comprehensive
- clear
- presented in a logical sequence
- with sufficient detail to inform the reader.

Several methods exist to present research data. This section offers you a range of examples that you may select from, as well as suggestions as to how they may be useful.

There are two commonly used methods for presenting data, namely tables and figures. Tables generally list literary information in block form, for example theoretical models, diagnostic criteria, common features of a problem, responses to a question and lists of percentages. Figures are used to illustrate data, for example diagrammatic representations of conceptual frameworks, flow charts and present information contained within a diagram. In addition to tables and figures, charts are also used to present data. Examples can be provided as follows:

- bar charts (horizontal, grouped, stacked, histograms and pyramids) – useful for presenting data which are concerned with comparative totals of numbers, proportions and ratios, as for instance mortality rates for road traffic accidents by age in a given year. Two histograms can be combined to form a pyramid, for example to illustrate data relating to population and gender
- pie charts – useful for comparing proportions such as the percentage of men and women that access primary healthcare services for well women and well men clinics
- scatterplots – useful to plot two variables, for example the frequency of cancer in a number of specific geographical areas
- line charts – are generally used for describing events over a period of time, for example the number of deaths from smoking in a county over a 20-year period.

Charts are a particularly useful method of presenting data, in that the impact of the data communicates proportions and ratio more clearly than if the same data were presented in table form. Charts also facilitate the use of colour so enabling the researcher to highlight both contrasts and common themes.

You will find references to useful guidelines for processing and presenting data in the further reading list, p. 122.

*Discussion, implications, limitations and recommendations*
In this part:

- there should be an analysis and discussion of the findings and their implications, for example for professional practice, research and education
- reference to the literature review and the aims of the study should be included in the critical analysis and discussion
- an appraisal of the overall strengths and limitations of the study should be undertaken
- recommendations for professional practice and further study should be made
- care should be taken that these do not go beyond the data arising from the study.

## Appendices

These should be clear and contain items which cannot be easily fitted into the text. Examples here include copies of the questionnaire used and copies of letters requesting permission to access subjects. Reference to all appendices should have been made in the main body of the report.

### References and bibliography

These should be listed separately and should be presented consistently using an appropriate referencing system such as Harvard or Vancouver. If you use such a format as this, the process of writing up becomes less daunting and it is possible to see how things fit together. It also allows you to divide the writing up into smaller, more manageable, units.

## Specific guidelines for dissertations by literature review

The review should consist of a comprehensive discussion and evaluation of the literature relating to an appropriate topic area within the course of study. The literature should be research based, and critiquing skills should be evident in the evaluation.

It would be helpful to choose a topic about which enough has been written to provide opportunities for critical analysis, otherwise the breadth and depth of the review will be limited.

*Note:* The general guidance outlined for dissertations involving data collection also applies to dissertations by literature review. Specific guidance regarding the main body of the review is outlined below.

### Introduction

This should include:

- background information on the topic reviewed and its relevance to practice, education or research, and the reasons for choosing the topic
- an explanation of any parameters set for the literature search, for example the last 15 years or British and American articles
- the aims and objectives of the review, together with an explanation and justification of the thematic progression of the subsequent chapters.

### The main body of the review

This should be arranged in logical progression according to the themes relating to the main topic. There is no set way to lay out the review, but it will be influenced by the topic you choose. Some reviews need to be organised under main chapter headings that facilitate the progression of the review. The main body of the review will usually include:

- discussion and analysis of the concepts and/or theories identified in the literature, which contribute to the knowledge and understanding of the topic
- critical analysis of the state and level of knowledge relating to the topic
- critical analysis of specific research reports, policy and professional documentation (some of which may be unpublished) relating to the aims of the study
- identification of gaps in the literature.

*Conclusion*

This should start with an overall summary of your review and then include:

- the implications of any limitations of your review, such as parameters not being sufficiently broad
- identification of implications and recommendations for professional practice, with an outline of how these can be incorporated into practice
- recommendations for future research.

# Producing a short report or executive summary from a main study

As highlighted earlier, the presentation of research is usually supported by short reports (500–600 words for example) so that the audience has a record of the key features of the work. The main subheadings are:

- title
- aims and objectives
- methodology
- main findings
- recommendations
- implications
- conclusions.

# Conclusion

It remains that the credibility of research activities relies on the thoroughness of each step of the process. The relationship between the problem or hypothesis, the aims of the study, the literature review and the methodology serve to justify how the main links for the research process have been operationalised.

This, in turn, underpins the quality of the analysis if the findings can be discussed in the light of all previous stages. Research activities often raise more questions than they answer, and this is to be expected. The outcomes of research activities are also depended upon, often when significant decisions are to be made, as for example in resourcing patient services or investment in new primary healthcare initiatives. The presentation of research is all-important and should always be as objective, precise and valid as possible.

The next section concludes the chapter and provides a step-by-step guide to the dissemination of research findings, including tips on presenting at a conference and getting published.

# Disseminating research outcomes

Most research projects have a valuable contribution to make to the knowledge base of the discipline concerned. Researchers who are new to this process commonly underestimate the value of their work and fail to disseminate the outcomes of their efforts appropriately. It is usually necessary to adapt an original report or dissertation for the purpose of a wider audience and often time is of the essence, particularly for topical subjects.

It is the responsibility of the researcher to ensure that the outcomes of a study are communicated effectively, which means preparing the work for local and/or national audiences. This task need not be undertaken in isolation, rather continuing to work on this with a project team or a suitable mentor will usually contribute to the overall sharing of the workload involved.

## Strategies for local dissemination of findings

Most healthcare research is intended for the public domain which means that the researcher needs to consider the method by which the outcome of the research is going to be presented to others. At a local level options can include:

- local specialist interest groups
- local newsletters and press
- in-house journals and magazines
- presentations at local meetings, professional groups
- delivering a report
- providing the information as a teaching session
- conducting a seminar as a part of a programme of study or course
- presenting the material at a research seminar
- local workshops and conferences.

*Exercise 2*

Consider your own role and place of work in primary care. Aim to identify outlets for disseminating findings from your research activity.

## Strategies for national and international dissemination of findings

As well as the local dissemination of research findings it is essential that as wide an audience as possible is reached for the findings of the research to have the desired impact on healthcare. This means in reality the presentation and/or publication of the material at national and possibly international level. It is important, however, that prior to the dissemination of the research findings at local, national and international level, permissions should have been sought and gained from all interested parties.

This includes the host organisation or institution in which the research was conducted and the agency funding the research. Equally, it is the responsibility of the researcher or research team to ensure that any ethical issues regarding the disclosure of information, particularly that which is of a sensitive nature or can be related to an individual, are resolved.

# Presentation

Presentation of the research material, usually at a conference, can take different forms:

- keynote address
- paper
- main session
- general session
- concurrent session
- plenary session
- special-interest group session
- seminar
- workshop
- poster session.

## Tips on presenting at a conference

When preparing to present at a conference there are several issues to consider:

- which group or groups of professionals do I want to present to? – determines the choice of the conference
- what funding is available or do I self-fund? – determines whether a national or international conference
- what format? – determines the amount and type of work required to prepare the material.

Once these issues have been worked through, scan the appropriate journals and magazines and look for calls for papers/contributors/presenters/participants. When you receive the information on the conference you will normally be given several options:

- a straightforward delivery of a paper to a static audience with limited feedback or delegate interaction, for example keynote address, main session, general session, concurrent session or plenary session
- the opportunity to present/contribute at the conference and try out teaching techniques or demonstrate research findings in an interactive way, by conducting a small-group workshop, seminar or specialist-interest group session

- the opportunity for participants to demonstrate or publicise their work in an exhibition area as a poster presentation.

It is also common practice for conference organisers to issue *abstract guidelines* for potential contributors to a conference and you will be expected to return some or all of the following information to the conference organiser:

- name
- job title/position
- previous presentation?
- workplace
- qualifications
- area of expertise
- mailing address
- telephone, fax and e-mail
- title of paper
- brief typed abstract or description of your proposed presentation
- choices of presentation style, e.g. paper, poster, etc.
- indicate which conference theme the material fits
- potential learning outcomes
- keywords
- reading list.

If your paper or presentation is accepted you will then be asked to:

- confirm attendance at the event
- provide biographical details for the conference programme/delegate pack
- confirm your requirements for presentation of the material, such as an overhead projector, slide projector, computer link-up, white board and so on
- provide details of your personal requirements such as diet, accommodation and access to buildings.

Once your work has been accepted for a conference it is important to consider the way in which the material will be presented and how you are going to prepare it for the event. Points to think about are:

- volume of information on each page, slide or poster
- using graphics and illustrations
- cartoons
- using different colours
- font, font style and font size
- using tables and figures
- presentation of statistics
- using pictures and drawings
- general layout.

# Publication

It is quite common for presentations at a conference to be published as a set of conference abstracts, conference papers or as some form of post-conference publication; however, the procedure and process for publishing a research article in a professional journal is different. Tips on getting published and some points that you will need to consider before starting the process are given below.

Publication of the research material takes different forms:

- abstract
- short report
- article
- chapter
- book.

# Tips on getting published

There is a large range of journals which publish primary healthcare articles. These include:

*British Journal of Community Nursing*
*British Journal of Midwifery*
*Community Practitioner*
*Health and Social Care in the Community*
*Health Informatics Journal*
*Journal of Health Services Research and Policy*
*Journal of Paediatric Nursing*
*Journal of Public Health Medicine*
*Practice Nurse*
*Primary Health Care*
*Public Health.*

In addition, a range of publishers promote primary healthcare publications. Useful addresses for such publishing houses include:

Arnold, 338 Euston Road, London NW1 3BH
Macmillan Press Ltd, Houndmills, Basingstoke, Hampshire RG21 6XS
Open University Press, 22 Ballmoor Court, Buckinghamshire MK18 1XW
Oxford University Press, Great Clarendon Street, Oxford OX2 6DP
Radcliffe Medical Press Ltd, 18 Marcham Road, Abingdon, Oxfordshire OX14 1AA
Routledge, 11 New Fetter Lane, London EC4P 4EE
Sage, 6 Bonhill Street, London EC2A 4PZ.

Whatever the form of publication, several questions and key points need to be addressed when working through the process of writing for publication.

- Who needs to know? – determines the type of audience to whom you wish to disseminate
- Who will be interested? – establishes the size of the audience
- How much do I want to say? – determines the length of the piece
- Which journal or publisher? – needs to be considered for marketing the piece
- What is the house style of the journal or publisher? – determines the style of presentation, therefore seek author guidelines.

The process of writing and successful publication of the results of a research project can take time. Publishing houses receive hundreds of articles every month and only a small percentage get published. A poor-quality paper is only one of several reasons why a publisher may not accept an article. Other reasons for articles not being accepted include:

- the editor may have commissioned an author to write an article that has a similar theme
- the editor may have already accepted an article that has a similar theme
- the journal may have just published (or has in press) an article of a similar theme
- journals generally work in cycles and may have a series of articles planned in the future which has a similar theme.

Therefore, before putting pen to paper or finger to keyboard:

- Search back through recent editions of the journal for articles which are similar to your own.
- Familiarise yourself with the style of the journal.
- Telephone or write to the editor of the journal you are considering submitting to and ask them if they are interested in your article.
- If yes, ask for guidelines for authors or house style in the case of a book and confirm verbally/in writing that you will be submitting an article to the journal and give a deadline date. If no, go back to the drawing board, don't get disheartened and ring the next editor on your list.
- Be prepared for your article not to be accepted by three or four journals before acceptance.
- Ask a colleague to read through your work and make constructive comments or seek out an editorial board member of a journal for their help.
- If your article is accepted and a review is asked for, don't give up, work on the article again and resubmit it.
- Be patient and tenacious.
- It is common practice for publishers to issue contracts for work being prepared for publication, therefore it is important to read through the conditions and deadlines set by the publisher.

All authors of research articles need help at the start of their experience.

## Conclusion

Now you have worked through this chapter, we hope you are able to use it for your own research activities in primary care and that you will take advantage of it again in the future as you take opportunities to produce research reports and disseminate outcomes.

Undertaking any research activity is a challenge but one which is essential if we are to continue to generate knowledge and understanding about what we do in primary healthcare. Research involving a range of members of the multidisciplinary team is to be encouraged, particularly as services and quality care depend on effective teamwork.

Writing up and presenting research is an all-important part of the research process and essential to its communication. Whether you produce an academic dissertation or a report, we hope the guidelines set out here have given you appropriate guidance.

# Answers to exercises

## Exercise 1

While there are a number of ways of organising and structuring a report or dissertation, which are explained in 'Contents of a written report', p. 109, having a clear vision of the intended contribution of the work to the field of practice is essential. There follows a range of perspectives which are pertinent to primary healthcare and which may be used to highlight, prioritise and add direction to the writing process. These include:

- policy and organisational responses to changes in healthcare needs
- the influence of health and social care reforms
- the impact of the internal market on primary healthcare
- involvement of the service user in collaborative initiatives
- care management and nursing initiatives, for example hospital at home
- the implications for general practice and the role of the practice nurse
- the implications for public health promotion and disease prevention.

## Exercise 2

As well as the options already listed, you may find relevant outlets through consumer groups, multidisciplinary forums and the voluntary and private sectors.

# References

Chapman H (1996) Why do nurses not make use of a solid research base? *Nursing Times*. **92**(3): 38–9.

Department of Health (1993) *Research for Health*. HMSO, London.

Department of Health (1994) *Supporting Research and Development in the NHS*. HMSO, London.

Department of Health and Social Security (1972) *Report of the Committee on Nursing*. Briggs Report. HMSO, London.

Edwards A and Talbot R (1994) *The Hard-pressed Researcher*. Longman, London.

Hicks C, Hennessy D, Cooper J *et al.* (1996) Investigating attitudes to research in primary health-care teams. *Journal of Advanced Nursing*. **24**: 1033–41.

Holm K and Llewellyn J G (1986) *Nursing Research for Nursing Practice*. W B Saunders and Company, Philadelphia.

McMahon A (1997) Implications for nursing of the NHS R&D funding policy. *Nursing Standard*. **11**(28): 44–8.

Marshall L and Rowland F (1993) *A Guide to Learning Independently*. Open University Press, Buckingham.

United Kingdom Central Council for Nursing, Midwifery and Health Visiting (1992) *Code of Professional Conduct for the Nurse, Midwife and Health Visitor* (3rd edn). UKCC, London.

# Further reading

Bell J (1993) *Doing Your Research Project*. Open University Press, Buckingham.

Blaxter L, Hughes C and Tight M (1996) *How to Research*. Open University Press, Buckingham.

Bowling A (1997) *Research Methods in Health: Investigating Health and Health Services*. Open University Press, Buckingham.

Couchman W and Davies J (1995) *Nursing and Health-care Research*. Scutari Press, London.

Crombie I K and Davies H T O (1996) *Research in Health Care*. John Wiley, Chichester.

Cryer P (1996) *The Research Student's Guide to Success*. Open University Press, Buckingham.

Hardey M and Mulhall A (eds) (1994) *Nursing Research – Theory and Practice*. Chapman and Hall, London.

Hart E and Bond M (1995) *Action Research for Health and Social Care*. Open University Press, Buckingham.

Hek G, Judd M and Moule P (1996) *Making Sense of Research*. Cassell, London.

Herbert M (1990) *Planning a Research Project*. Cassell, London.

McNiff J, Lomax P and Whitehead J (1996) *You and Your Action Research Project*. Routledge, London.

Nortledge A (1994) *The Good Study Guide*. The Open University, Milton Keynes.

Polgar S and Thomas S A (1995) *Introduction to Research in the Health Sciences*. Churchill Livingstone, Melbourne.

Popay J and Williams G (1994) *Researching the People's Health*. Routledge, London.

Shakespeare P, Atkinson D and French S (1993) *Reflecting on Research Practice*. Open University Press, Buckingham.

Smith P (ed) (1997) *Research-mindedness for Practice*. Churchill Livingstone, London.

Wallgren A, Wallgren B, Persson R *et al.* (1996) *Graphing Statistics and Data*. Sage Publications, California.

# CHAPTER SIX

# Implementing research findings

*Richard Baker*

## Introduction

Primary healthcare teams are increasingly required to base their practice on evidence and to use effective methods of implementing research findings. The aim of this chapter is to introduce the main principles relevant to primary healthcare teams that want to implement research findings. Several simple exercises are included, but there are also some more advanced excrcises for those who wish to investigate the topic in greater detail or consider research into the subject. The exercises will help the reader to become familiar with the tasks involved in finding and implementing research evidence. There are no right answers to the exercises and so none are suggested.

The detailed objectives of the chapter are that, as a result of considering its contents, the primary healthcare team will be:

- aware of sources of good-quality summaries of research evidence
- able to undertake simple appraisals of sources of evidence
- able to investigate the potential obstacles that might face implementation of particular research findings by the team
- able to design and put into practice effective strategies to implement research findings.

Recently, few topics have occupied the minds of health service policy makers and academics, or filled so many pages of health service journals, as the challenge of improving the effectiveness of clinical care. The NHS Executive went so far as to create a specific initiative, to which it gave the name of clinical effectiveness (NHS Management Executive 1993). The aim was to encourage better use of research evidence, and initially the core of the initiative was advice to purchasers to base their decisions on the best available evidence. They were to concentrate their resources on care shown to be effective and reduce expenditure on care shown to be relatively ineffective. Concerns such as these have now become familiar to practice teams, especially fundholders. The clinical-effectiveness programme has since expanded to include systems to support the development of evidence-based guidelines and most recently the creation of a national organisation to appraise guidelines so that they can be recommended to those working in the NHS. A framework for linking clinical audit and other activities that support clinical effectiveness has also been put forward (NHS Executive 1996).

Of course, changing clinical practice is rarely easy, whether the changes involve the way individual practitioners perform or, on a broader level, the agreement of purchasing policies. In recognition of these problems, a specific section of the NHS Research and Development Programme was established in order to identify more effective methods of implementing research findings. It will be several years before the results of the studies commissioned in this programme are available, but even so further research is needed. Therefore, if you are considering becoming involved in research, the topic of implementing change deserves some thought. In particular, we need more information about methods appropriate for the multidisciplinary teams typical of primary healthcare.

It is not only primary healthcare teams that have come across this preoccupation with improving the effectiveness of care by basing it on convincing research evidence. Many specialties have begun to develop clinical guidelines that have apparently been derived from evidence. In the clinical journals, emphasis is increasingly being placed on the quality of research evidence and on explaining to readers how to appraise that evidence. Continuing education for team members has begun to reflect the same themes. Perhaps the most powerful influence has been the evidence-based medicine movement. This has the aim of training practitioners, whether they be nurses, doctors or other health professionals, to make conscientious, explicit and judicious use of current best evidence in making decisions about the care of individual patients (Sackett *et al.* 1997). Its arrival in the UK has been followed by the emergence of numerous enthusiastic followers. Evidence-based medicine argues that each clinician should have the skills to appraise reports of research and implement the findings if appropriate. The skills can be difficult to acquire, the jargon can be confusing and it is not surprising that some clinicians have viewed the arrival of evidence-based medicine with suspicion.

# The problems

Many teams will have had experiences similar to that described in Box 6.1. The first problem is the inexorable flow of new research and new recommendations about the way we should provide care. It is now impossible for any health professional to read all the relevant research published in his or her discipline. We need new ways of finding information about research and keeping up to date.

The second problem is that even if we were able to read all the latest evidence, changing performance is far from simple. The danger of repeated failure to implement change is that a sense of impotence will be generated. The team will become unwilling in the future to try to change performance unless there is a major incentive or substantial

---

**Box 6.1** An example of failed implementation in one primary healthcare team

The primary care team cared for a patient population of just over 11 000 patients, most of whom lived in the suburbs of a large town. There were five general practitioners, a practice manager, four practice nurses, five attached nurses, a practice counsellor and physiotherapist. It had been a training practice for more than 15 years. After a team meeting on Friday lunch-time there was a feeling of disappointment. A year ago they had undertaken the first part of an audit of diabetes care. The findings from their data collection made clear that improvements were required. Patients were not being seen regularly, the level of their diabetes control was not being checked and routine examinations for signs of complications were often omitted. That Friday, the results of the second data collection had been presented and there had been no improvement. Despite all the good intentions and acceptance that research evidence had shown that improved management of patients with diabetes could reduce the risk of long-term complications, the team had failed to make any progress.

This had not been their first experience of failure. Two years ago they had attempted to improve asthma care but had been unsuccessful. At that same Friday meeting, the team noted that it had been invited to take part in a local scheme to improve the proportion of patients with coronary heart disease risk factors who were taking aspirin. In view of their past experiences, they were unable to face taking part in yet another attempt to implement research that they believed would be doomed to fail.

---

external help. In fact, such pessimism is often unjustified. We change our clinical behaviour more frequently than we realise, even if there is often delay between being informed of new research findings and eventual change in practice. Teams are also subject to influence by others seeking to change clinical practice, for example health service managers, academics, educators and pharmaceutical companies. These agents use a variety of methods, from advertising to complex educational techniques, and may include financial incentives or sanctions. Evidently, there are methods that can be used to implement research findings – perhaps we could use these ourselves.

# Finding the evidence

Suppose in our example that someone in the team points out that aspirin was thought to be an effective intervention for reducing the risk of death in patients who had a history of myocardial infarction. However, another member of the team said they thought the benefits of aspirin were not all that impressive. One of the partners, Dr Benedict, was delegated to find evidence to resolve this difference of opinion.

She went to the local university where the librarian advised her to look for information in the Cochrane Library on CD-ROM. She followed this advice and found a detailed review that provided the information needed by the team. If you are not familiar with the Cochrane Library, complete Exercise 1.

*Exercise 1*

1.  Locate a copy of the Cochrane Library – it is on CD-ROM and should be available, for example, at your local postgraduate centre library. Some practices also subscribe to the Cochrane Library. It is published four times per year, and details on the Internet can be found at *http://www.cochrane.co.uk.*

2.  Load the Library on your PC, click on Search and opt for the simple format. Type in 'aspirin'. In the third issue of the 1997 volume of the Library there were no Cochrane reviews of the effectiveness of aspirin as secondary prevention after myocardial infarction. However, the review found by Dr Benedict is listed in the abstracts of reviews of effectiveness, also included on the CD. Read the abstract of the Antiplatelet Trialists' Collaboration (1994).

3.  What are the conclusions of the reviews of aspirin and stroke? Should Dr Benedict recommend to her team that they advise patients who have had a stroke to take aspirin?

4.  Try a more complex search using the Cochrane Library, for example 'aspirin *and* myocardial infarction'.

The review found by Dr Benedict was undertaken by the Antiplatelet Trialists' Collaboration (1994). At first sight it looked like a heavy read, but the Cochrane abstract and the abstract of the review itself both made the important message clear. In patients with a past history of myocardial infarction, treatment with aspirin 75–325 mg/day for two years would prevent 40 vascular events (non-fatal myocardial infarctions, non-fatal strokes and vascular deaths) for every 1000 patients. Of the 40 events prevented, 24 on average would be vascular deaths. Thus, to prevent one event the practice would have to treat 25 patients for two years (or 50 patients for one year). To prevent one death, they would have to treat 41 patients for two years. These figures, sometimes referred to as the 'numbers needed to treat' (NNT – see Sackett *et al.* 1997, page 133, for further information), compare well with other interventions such as control of hypertension, or treatment of acute myocardial infarction with streptokinase. Therefore, the team agreed that the benefit from secondary prevention with aspirin was worthwhile.

# MEDLINE

An alternative way to find systematic reviews is to use one of the established electronic bibliographic databases. The most accessible and widely used is MEDLINE. It contains an enormous number of references, but has a North American bias. EMBASE is an alternative that has a greater proportion of European publications. MEDLINE is available in most medical libraries, and British Medical Association (BMA) members can use it from their home computers through an Internet connection. Because it is a complex database, there are several software packages that can be used to search MEDLINE. Exercise 2 shows the use of the OVID package to search MEDLINE through an Internet connection to the BMA.

## Exercise 2

The use of MEDLINE to find systematic reviews of aspirin in secondary prevention of myocardial infarction.

1.  Find a convenient point of access to MEDLINE. If you are unsure where to start, contact your local medical/university library.
2.  Log on to OVID and use the 1993–1997 MEDLINE database. You will be asked to enter search statements, one at a time. When you press <enter> after each line, the database is searched to find the relevant articles. By combining the searches, you can locate relevant articles.
3.  Box 6.2 shows a search that was undertaken in September 1997 to seek systematic reviews on the effectiveness of aspirin as secondary prevention. Try this search out and see what you find.

---

**Box 6.2**  Example of a search undertaken to seek systematic reviews on the effectiveness of aspirin as secondary prevention

| Line number | Entry | Number of articles |
|---|---|---|
| 1 | meta-analysis.sh. | 917 |
| 2 | meta-analy$.tw. | 2088 |
| 3 | metaanal$.tw. | 108 |
| 4 | meta-analysis.pt. | 1786 |
| 5 | ((systematic$ adj4 (review$ or overview$)).tw. | 517 |
| 6 | exp review literature/ | 366 |
| 7 | or/1-6 | 3908 |
| 8 | animal.sh. | 503 776 |
| 9 | human.sh. | 1 191 917 |
| 10 | 9 not 8 | 1 055 211 |
| 11 | 7 and 10 | 3570 |
| 12 | aspirin$.tw. | 3241 |
| 13 | platelet$.tw. | 19 410 |
| 14 | antiplatelet$.tw. | 1069 |
| 15 | or/12-14 | 22 366 |
| 16 | myocardial infarction.tw. | 11 826 |
| 17 | infarct$.tw. | 18 829 |
| 18 | or/16-17 | 18 829 |
| 19 | 11 and 15 | 81 |
| 20 | 18 and 19 | 26 |

*Key*
tw. – textword
$ – covers all possible extensions to the preceding word, for example plurals
pt. – publication type, e.g. reviews, RCTs, etc.
sh. – MeSH heading
adj4 – within four words

The first six lines select the type of studies to be included, in this case systematic reviews. Line 7 brings these six lines together. Next, studies with animal subjects are eliminated, and the remainder combined with the reviews (line 11). Then the subject of the reviews we want to find is entered, first aspirin therapy (lines 12–15) then myocardial infarction (16–18). Note that the term 'infarct$.tw.' identified all articles of line 16 plus some additional articles.

Twenty-six articles were found. On scrolling through the abstracts on screen, the Antiplatelet Trialists' Collaboration (1994) review was included, but there were also some other useful references. There was a paper giving guidance to general practitioners about how to respond to the findings of this important review (Moher and Lancaster 1996). Another review considered the appropriate dose of aspirin (Patrono and Roth 1996). Although a dose of 75–160 mg was effective in patients with a history of cardiovascular disease, there was some doubt about the dose for those with a history of cerebrovascular disease. The review recommended use of the present low-dose schedule, but thought that this advice might be changed depending on the results of future definitive studies.

Can you undertake a MEDLINE search for randomised controlled trials of aspirin in secondary prevention? Some useful advice can be found in Sackett *et al.* (1997).

## Systematic reviews

A systematic review (sometimes called an overview) provided the guidance for our example primary healthcare team. An increasing number of such reviews is becoming available and generally they can be recommended as a safer alternative to obtaining evidence directly from individual studies. Of course, reviews of the literature have been available for many years, but the systematic review is different in several important respects. In particular, explicit methods are used to identify, appraise and synthesise the findings from different studies. These techniques reduce the risk of conclusions being biased by the personal views of the authors.

In a systematic review, the steps taken to identify all relevant studies must be described. First, several electronic bibliographic databases will have been searched (for example MEDLINE, EMBASE, CINAHL), as no single database is comprehensive. To supplement these searches, the authors may follow up references in the papers they find, or hand-search selected journals, or contact experts to ask for information about unpublished studies. If such methods are not used, there is a danger that important evidence will be overlooked.

Second, when the studies have been identified they must be assessed for quality. If poor-quality trials are used in the review, the conclusions may well be wrong. Often the effect of poor-quality studies is to exaggerate the effectiveness of the treatment being investigated. The majority of reviews limit the included studies to randomised controlled trials, although even then the quality of these must be assessed (Guyatt *et al.* 1993).

In the third main stage of a systematic review, the included studies are brought together to produce an overall finding. If the studies involve relatively similar types of patient receiving relatively similar treatments, and the trial designs are similar, it may be possible to combine the original data. This is called meta-analysis. The review of aspirin therapy used this approach (Antiplatelet Trialists' Collaboration 1994). However, sometimes it is not possible to combine data from different studies and the only alternative is to describe the findings without any mathematical analysis. This approach is referred to as a qualitative analysis.

In the same way that particular research studies can have weaknesses, some systematic reviews can also be criticised. Because the most appropriate methods for systematic reviews have been established, it is possible for the quality of reviews to be appraised. Simple appraisal methods are available and if you have doubts about a review it would be wise to apply these before deciding whether to accept or reject the conclusions (Oxman *et al.* 1994; Oxman and Guyatt 1988).

### *Exercise 3*

Read the paper in the *Journal of the American Medical Association* series 'Users' guides to the medical literature' about systematic reviews (Oxman *et al.* 1994). Use the advice about appraising reviews to assess a systematic review of steroid injections for shoulder disorders (van der Heijden *et al.* 1996). What are your conclusions?

## Clinical practice guidelines

Guidelines offer another source of summaries of research evidence. However, the quality of guidelines is variable and many have not been developed from research evidence but are merely the informal distillation of opinions and prejudices of their developers. However, guidelines do have the advantage that they can address the complete management of a major condition that could not be considered in a single systematic review. When evidence is limited, they can combine it with opinion to produce recommendations that may be helpful.

Different methods can be used to develop guidelines, and some methods lead to guidelines that are best ignored. However, when appropriate methods are used, guidelines can be helpful in clinical practice. The guidelines to avoid are those that have been developed through informal consensus. These rely on the authority of the guideline panel, and in essence they are instructing clinicians to do what they are told. This approach would be acceptable if we could be confident that the recommendations of the panel are sound. Unfortunately, this is not always the case; and even when the recommendations are probably correct, the potential user is unable to verify this because the guideline does not make reference to evidence.

The best guidelines are evidence based, that is, they make explicit links between the recommendations they contain and the underlying research (Royal College of General Practitioners 1995). This type of guideline does not rely on the authority of the panel. Because the evidence leading to the recommendations is explained, the guideline user can check whether he or she agrees. The documentation should include full details of the literature search that was undertaken, how the quality of studies was appraised and a date by which the guideline should be regarded as expired. Thus, guidelines may be based on one or several systematic literature reviews. However, in addition to drawing on several reviews, guidelines try to address the problem of variable evidence. Since the strength of evidence will depend on the number and quality of relevant studies, recommendations are accompanied by indication of the strength of the supporting evidence.

Unfortunately, evidence is sometimes very limited. In these circumstances the guideline panel has to fall back on its own opinions, and therefore these recommendations are open to the same criticisms that are levelled against consensus guidelines. However, by making clear which recommendations are supported by evidence and which by opinion, clinical judgement rather than blind obedience can be employed by the guideline user when caring for patients.

Because guidelines are of variable quality, it is wise to critically assess a guideline before you decide to accept its recommendations. Standard methods for appraising guidelines are available (Cluzeau *et al.* 1995; Hayward *et al.* 1995). To explore this process further, undertake Exercise 4.

*Exercise 4*

Obtain a copy of Hayward *et al.* (1995). Apply this guideline assessment method to two guidelines. One guideline should be the North of England guideline on asthma (North of England Guidance Development Group 1996). This is an example of a systematically developed, evidence-based guideline for general practice. Choose the second guideline yourself. If possible, this should be a locally developed guideline for the same or related topic. Which guideline do you think provides the most valid advice?

# Other sources of information

Most of us regularly read, or scan, some journals relevant to our discipline. However, it is impossible to remain up to date no matter how obsessional we may be at studying journals. We need someone to do much of our reading for us, and to meet this need two journals have been launched that contain abstracts of key papers from the world literature. *ACP Journal Club* and *Evidence-based Medicine* are published quarterly and are available in most postgraduate libraries. *Bandolier* is a less formal journal that also occasionally includes summaries of evidence. A disadvantage of these journals is that they address the needs of all clinical specialties and therefore cannot meet in detail the needs of an individual specialty.

Many other sources of information about evidence are becoming available. Most regional offices of the NHS have set up systems for appraising evidence in order to advise purchasers. For example, in Trent, purchasers, including primary healthcare teams, identify topics. Experts are commissioned to undertake reviews which are studied by a regional Development and Evaluation Committee, which then issues guidance. Information about these reports and how to obtain them is published in various regional newsletters, but an easy way to find out more about them is to contact the regional office Internet web sites. You can also find web sites devoted to particular conditions, although some of these are operated by vested interests and the evidence they recommend may be both limited and biased.

In this chapter, the identification and assessment of primary studies such as randomised controlled trials has not been discussed. This requires more time and more expertise, and good-quality summaries of evidence should be used when possible. However, if you wish to find out more about finding and appraising trials, study relevant articles in the 'Users' guide' series in the *Journal of the American Medical Association*, or refer to Sackett *et al.* (1997).

# Implementing the evidence

In recent years there have been many research studies of methods of implementing the findings of research. The studies have included doctors in primary and secondary care, nurses and other health professionals, and they have been asked to implement all manner of clinical activities. The randomised controlled trial is the most reliable study design for providing information about these types of interventions to change clinical performance. Because experiments on behaviours such as clinical performance are so liable to be at risk from bias from unwanted effects, sometimes called 'Hawthorn' effects, randomised controlled trials are to be preferred. Although they are not altogether free from bias, they do minimise the potential problems. Should the primary healthcare team described in Box 6.3 search for randomised controlled trials of methods of implementing change? They could, but this would be an inefficient use of their time. In addition, they may not possess the skills to appraise the quality of individual trials and may be at risk of drawing false conclusions. A more sensible approach would be for them to seek good-quality systematic reviews.

---

**Box 6.3**     The primary healthcare team seeks information on implementation

Our primary care team had accepted that aspirin therapy was indicated for the secondary prevention of myocardial infarction and other vascular events. In view of their past experiences of failure to implement the findings of research, they wanted more information about the methods they could use that would be more likely to be effective. Because Dr Benedict had been so successful at finding evidence about the effectiveness of aspirin, she was delegated to find information about possible implementation methods.

She went back to the library and once again consulted the Cochrane Library. Several reviews looked promising. She printed out a Cochrane review of the effectiveness of printed educational materials (Freemantle *et al.* 1997) and asked the librarian for photocopies of two reviews (Davis *et al.* 1995; Grimshaw *et al.* 1995).

The systematic reviews found by Dr Benedict provide a useful starting point for considering methods of implementing research findings. The total number of good-quality trials of implementation methods is now large, and it is possible to draw some general conclusions. However, the number of studies of any individual method is still relatively small and much work remains to be done.

Two factors appear to be important. First, if the implementation method operates during the interaction between patient and professional it is more likely to be effective. Thus, reminder systems, such as computer prompts or records that are structured to promote particular clinical actions, can be effective. Conversely, reminders that are distant from the consultation, such as general reminders before clinics, are less effective, and written educational materials often have little effect.

Second, implementation methods that more actively involve the health professional tend to be more effective. For example, traditional passive educational methods, such as lectures or seminars, are relatively ineffective, but those requiring active participation, such as academic detailing methods, are more effective. The effectiveness of feedback generally falls between these two, but is more effective if it provides information about the personal performance of the targeted individual rather than the performance of the team as a whole. An outline of the methods and their effectiveness is shown in Table 6.1.

Unfortunately, the choice of implementation method cannot rely on picking those that appear more effective. In addition to showing that some methods appear more effective, the available studies also show that no single method is invariably effective. On different occasions, in different settings, any method can fail. No single method can be relied upon to bring about changes in clinical practice. Because the impact of implementation methods is difficult to predict, Wensing and Grol (1994) have suggested that the use of two

**Table 6.1** Implementation methods and their effectiveness

| Implementation methods | Evidence of effectiveness |
| --- | --- |
| Feedback, e.g. as in audit | General feedback – less effective<br>Personal feedback – more effective |
| Reminders – paper or computer | During consultations – more effective<br>Distant from consultations – less effective |
| Opinion leaders | Variable effectiveness – more evidence is needed |
| Facilitation | Appears appropriate for primary healthcare teams but little evidence is available |
| Patient-mediated interventions, e.g. patient reminders | Relatively effective but may be practical for only a limited range of topics, e.g. routine health checks |
| Conferences | Little or no effect |
| Educational materials, e.g. guidelines | Little or no effect unless accompanied by other strategies |
| Academic detailing | Relatively effective – but more evidence is needed about the range of topics that can be addressed |
| Total quality management | Little information available |
| Reorganisation of services | Probably relatively effective although more evidence would be helpful |
| Advertising | Relatively few studies – effectiveness therefore uncertain |

methods simultaneously would increase the reliability of efforts to implement research findings.

An alternative approach to this problem is to attempt to understand the factors that make change more or less likely. We have suggested a framework for addressing this problem that has similarities with making a clinical assessment of a patient (Robertson *et al.* 1996). In different settings, when research findings are implemented, different obstacles to change may be present. These may be caused by the organisation of the health service, limitations of the primary healthcare team or because of characteristics of individuals in the team. Depending on the cause of the obstacles, different implementation methods will be more effective. For example, providing feedback when the obstacle to change is lack of resources in the organisation will have little effect, and may only lead to a loss of morale among professionals.

The obstacles may be regarded as the symptoms of the underlying problem. When presented with symptoms and signs, the clinician relates them to possible diseases, and for each disease there is a particular treatment. In the case of implementing change, a behavioural scientist may think of the diseases as psychological or put forward other theories explaining human behaviour. However, in managing a primary healthcare team, a pragmatic approach would be more practical. An analysis of the obstacles to change might include an assessment of the educational needs of team members, investigation of the systems of work such as appointment intervals, or review of the structure of clinical records. Implementation methods can then be selected to match the findings of the analysis. This process will be discussed further later in the chapter, but first more information is given about some implementation methods.

# Audit

Audit will be familiar to all primary healthcare teams and several excellent introductory books are available (see for example, Irvine and Irvine 1997). Therefore, only a few key points will be mentioned here. Audit has five principal steps:

(1)   choice of topic
(2)   specification of desired performance in terms of criteria and standards
(3)   first data collection
(4)   implementation of change
(5)   second data collection.

The first point is to emphasise the importance of collecting data for the second time after changes have been implemented. Because no implementation method can be relied upon, it is essential to assess their impact, and use additional methods if necessary. The second point is that the criteria and standards play a crucial role as they depend on the research evidence. The selection of criteria is too often an informal consensus process, depending on the opinions and strength of voices of the participants rather than an explicit critical review of the literature. The principles for developing criteria have been described (Baker and Fraser 1995), and standard evidence-based criteria are available and have been shown to be acceptable (Baker and Fraser 1997). When used in audit, criteria of this type, which have been derived from evidence and prioritised according to the strength of evidence and impact on outcome, are more likely to promote benefits in care.

In trials of the effectiveness of audit in implementing change, the focus of attention has usually been feedback. The findings suggest that feedback can be effective, although to a variable extent. However, feedback is only one method that can be used in audit, as all the other methods may be used. Thus, audit should be regarded as the process for assessing the need for, and impact of, implementation methods. It is a fundamental feature of the clinical management of change.

## Academic detailing

Detailing is a marketing technique in which a sales person visits the target customer. In the pharmaceutical industry the sales representative is also known as a 'detailer' (Zikmund and d'Amico 1996). In adapting this method, emphasis has been placed on educating the target health professional, and therefore it has also been referred to as 'educational outreach' (Soumerai and Avorn 1990).

The objectives of the visit must be established beforehand, and some preliminary market research is undertaken to identify the issues that are likely to be important to the target professionals. During the visit the detailer explores the professional's current understanding of the topic and offers information required to fill the gaps in knowledge or to change opinions. Active learner involvement is sought, key messages are repeated and simple graphical materials are left with the professional as reinforcement.

The effectiveness of academic detailing has been investigated in trials of prescribing (Wayne *et al.* 1986; Avorn *et al.* 1992) and appropriateness of blood transfusions (Soumerai *et al.* 1993). The findings indicate that it is an effective approach, but its applicability in primary healthcare in the UK has yet to be established. In one study an intervention combining educational outreach with team facilitation methods was effective in implementing guidelines for diabetes and asthma (Feder *et al.* 1995). Other trials of this method are now being undertaken. Among the questions that remain to be answered are whether a member of a team can act as a detailer to colleagues in the same team, and whether the method is effective for implementing complex clinical behaviours such as diagnostic skills rather than only discrete, more simple behaviours such as prescribing.

## Opinion leaders

The decisions of consumers are influenced by other people in the social groups to which the consumer belongs. Such groups might be clubs, families or colleagues at work. Groups often include individuals who have particular influence because they are regarded as having expertise or respected personal attributes (Zikmund and d'Amico 1996). Although health professionals are taught to apply research evidence in their clinical practice, they are not immune to the influence of colleagues, and interest has grown in methods of directing this influence to control changes in performance.

The concept of social influence arises from research in the disciplines of psychology and sociology. We are all liable to be influenced by the norms of the social environment. This influence may take place in different settings: either in one-to-one interactions between individuals, or in groups or through mass media. Opinion leaders may be able to change the prevailing norms of a group of professionals. The methods for using opinion leaders to change clinical practice may vary, but generally rely on providing the selected leader with information about the research evidence and then leaving them to choose whatever approach they feel is appropriate to their setting (Lomas 1994).

Some information is available about the effectiveness of opinion leaders in implementing changes in performance (Davis *et al.* 1995; Grimshaw *et al.* 1995). Although this does suggest the method can be effective, its effect is not always reliable. We do not yet have sufficient knowledge to make firm recommendations about its use in primary healthcare. For example, the characteristics of typical opinion leaders are uncertain, the factors that govern the match between team characteristics and types of opinion leader are unclear and whether opinion leaders in their own teams can play roles in implementation is not known. The concept of opinion leaders is also rather confused. If an opinion leader is not effective, he or she has not led opinion and cannot be called an 'opinion leader'. This makes it difficult to define, identify and research the effectiveness of this approach.

# Reminders

There is a good deal of information available about the effectiveness of reminders (Davis *et al.* 1995; Grimshaw *et al.* 1995). This should confirm that reminders that operate in consultations are more effective, although invariably this is not the case (Baker *et al.* 1997). Nevertheless, computerised reminder systems are attracting much attention as an implementation method that might be widely used in the future. Even so, many research questions remain to be addressed. These include the most appropriate consultation techniques to ensure that the reminder is blended with the natural flow of the patient–professional interaction rather than being imposed and therefore having a distorting effect. With the growing attention being given to involving patients in decision making, we need new ways to balance the demands of evidence-based practice with patient preferences. This implies more detailed investigation of consultation and communication skills.

# Teamwork

There is surprisingly little evidence about the influence of teamwork on the implementation of research findings. We know that teamwork in primary healthcare is often deficient and that some teams offer more developed services than others, but the more common obstacles facing teams are not described, and how such obstacles might be overcome is uncertain. The majority of the implementation methods that have been investigated relate to the performance of individual professionals, or occasionally unidisciplinary groups of either doctors or nurses (see Table 6.1).

Practice managers may have a role to play. There is some evidence that the reorganisation of systems of work, or the allocation of tasks to multidisciplinary groups, can lead to change (Yano *et al.* 1995). However, the research evidence is limited. Whilst practice managers are integral to the team, facilitators are external, being brought in to support the team for short periods. During the last decade the number of facilitators working with health authorities and audit groups has increased steeply. There is some evidence about the effectiveness of facilitators in implementing change (Baker and Hearnshaw 1997), but once again the available evidence is limited. Evidently, there is no shortage of potential topics for those wishing to undertake research into methods of implementing research in primary care.

# A framework

The key to selecting a method for implementing research is to identify the particular obstacles to change and to match these with appropriate methods. A team can use several methods for identifying the obstacles:

- *audit* – the collection of data about current performance will show where the deficiencies lie and how much remains to be achieved. This is essential information for targeting efforts
- *brainstorming* – the team itself will have ideas about the problems. The use of systematic methods such as brainstorming will allow the majority of possible obstacles to be identified
- *cause and effect diagrams* – the detailed analysis of a process (for example a diabetic clinic) can help to reveal the causes of problems. The cause and effect diagram, or fish-bone chart, is a useful way of helping the team think through what the causes might be (Oakland 1993)
- *interviews* – confidential interviews with team members will enable the personal concerns and individual attitudes to emerge. An invited external facilitator may undertake the interviews. An alternative approach might be confidential questionnaires.

Having identified the obstacles, methods must be selected. Those that are most likely to be practical for a primary healthcare team include educational meetings for team members, reminder systems including revised records, feedback, or changes to systems of work such as clinics. Having applied one or more of these methods, the degree of success should be checked by audit. It would appear that implementing research is a process that has to be managed rather than left to chance or the personal preoccupations of team members. Now try Exercises 5 and 6.

*Exercise 5*

Implementation of aspirin in secondary prevention.

1.   Reread the description of the primary care team in Box 6.1.
2.   Write down the possible obstacles facing this team in implementing research about aspirin in secondary prevention of myocardial infarction. Because few details of the team are included, speculate – what obstacles might be present in your own team?
3.   Select implementation methods to overcome the obstacles.
4.   Repeat the exercise for a recent effort to implement research findings in your own team.

*Exercise 6*

Implementation methods for primary healthcare teams.

1.   Obtain copies of Davis *et al.* (1995) and Grimshaw *et al.* (1995). Study these systematic reviews.
2.   Identify those methods that would be practical for a primary healthcare team to employ.
3.   What assistance would a team need to use some of the other methods?

# Research points

There are many questions about the implementation of research that need to be addressed. They are too numerous to list here. The need for further studies relevant to primary healthcare has been a recurrent theme in this chapter. Both exploratory, qualitative studies and formal randomised controlled trials are required. If you are thinking of research in this field, it may be helpful to discuss your ideas with a behavioural scientist as progress will be more likely if studies are linked to theories of human behaviour.

# Conclusions

The implementation of research is often regarded as difficult. However, this chapter has suggested that there are practical methods that can be used in primary care. The first step is to find the evidence, and when possible summaries of evidence should be preferred to interminable, detailed literature searches. Let others more familiar with the techniques and with more time available do this work.

There are many implementation methods. The choice between them depends on the particular obstacles to change that are present and the evidence about the effectiveness of different methods. Teams can select methods themselves following investigation of the obstacles they face. Effective implementation therefore relies on systematic management that is supported by clinical audit.

# References

Antiplatelet Trialists' Collaboration (1994) Collaborative overview of randomised trials of antiplatelet therapy. I: Prevention of death, myocardial infarction, and stroke by prolonged antiplatelet therapy in various categories of patients. *British Medical Journal.* **308**: 81–106.

Avorn J, Soumerai S B, Everitt M D *et al.* (1992) Randomized trial of a program to reduce the use of psychoactive drugs in nursing homes. *New England Journal of Medicine.* **327**: 168–73.

Baker R and Fraser R C (1995) Development of review criteria: linking guidelines and assessment of quality. *British Medical Journal.* **311**: 370–3.

Baker R, Farooqi A, Tait C and Walsh S (1997) Randomised controlled trial of reminders to enhance the impact of audit in general practice on management of patients who use benzodiazepines. *Quality in Health Care.* **6**: 14–18.

Baker R and Fraser R C (1997) Is ownership more important than the scientific credibility of audit protocols? A survey of medical audit advisory groups. *Family Practice.* **14**: 107–11.

Baker R and Hearnshaw H (1997) Multidisciplinary clinical audit and primary healthcare teams. In: J Spencer and P Pearson (eds) *Promoting Teamwork in Primary Care.* Arnold, London.

Cluzeau F, Littlejohns P, Grimshaw J and Feder G (1995) Draft guideline appraisal tool. In: *The Development and Implementation of Clinical Guidelines.* Report from practice 26. RCGP, London.

Davis D A, Thomson M A, Oxman A D and Haynes R B (1995) Changing physician performance: a systematic review of the effect of continuing medical education strategies. *Journal of the American Medical Association.* **274**: 700–5.

Feder G, Griffths C, Highton C *et al.* (1995) Do clinical guidelines introduced with practice-based education improve care of asthmatic and diabetic patients? A randomised controlled trial in general practices in East London. *British Medical Journal.* **311**: 1473–8.

Freemantle N, Harvey E L, Grimshaw J M *et al.* (1997) The effectiveness of printed educational materials in improving the behaviour of health professionals and outcomes. In: L Bero, R Grilli, J Grimshaw *et al.* (eds) *Collaboration on Effective Professional Practice Module of The Cochrane Database of Systematic Reviews.* Available in The Cochrane Library. The Cochrane Collaboration: issue 1. Update Software, Oxford.

Grimshaw J, Freemantle N, Wallace S *et al.* (1995) Developing and implementing clinical practice guidelines. *Quality in Health Care.* **4**: 55–64.

Guyatt G H, Sackett D L, Cook D J for the Evidence-based Medicine Working Group (1993) Users' guides to the medical literature. II. How to use an article about therapy or prevention. A. Are the results valid? *Journal of the American Medical Association.* **270**: 2598–601.

Hayward R S A, Wilson M C, Tunis S R *et al.* for the Evidence-based Medicine Working Group (1995) Users' guides to the medical literature. VIII. How to use clinical practice guidelines. A. Are the recommendations valid? *Journal of the American Medical Association.* **274**: 570–4.

Institute of Medicine (1992) *Guidelines for Clinical Practice: From Development to Use* (eds M J Field and K N Lohr). National Academy Press, Washington, DC.

Irvine D and Irvine S (eds) (1997) *Making Sense of Audit* (2nd edn). Radcliffe Medical Press, Oxford.

Lomas J (1994) Teaching old (and not so old) docs new tricks: effective ways to implement research findings. In: E V Dunn, P G Norton, M Stewart *et al.* (eds) *Disseminating Research/ Changing Practice.* Sage Publications, Thousand Oaks.

Moher M and Lancaster T (1996) Who needs antiplatelet therapy? *British Journal of General Practice.* **46**: 367–70.

NHS Executive (1996) *Promoting Clinical Effectiveness: a framework for action in and through the NHS.* NHS Executive, London.

NHS Management Executive (1993) *Improving clinical effectiveness.* EL(93)115. Department of Health, Leeds.

North of England Asthma Guideline Development Group (1996) North of England Evidence-based Guidelines Development Project: summary version of evidence-based guidelines for the primary care management of asthma in adults. *British Medical Journal.* **312**: 762–6.

Oakland J (1993) *Total Quality Management: The Route to Improving Performance* (2nd edn). Butterworth Heinemann, Oxford.

Oxman A D and Guyatt G H (1988) Guidelines for reading literature reviews. *Canadian Medical Association Journal.* **138**: 697–703.

Oxman A D, Cook D J, Guyatt G H for the Evidence-based Medicine Working Group (1994) Users' guides to the medical literature. VI. How to use an overview. *Journal of the American Medical Association.* **272**: 1367–71.

Patrono C and Roth G J (1996) Aspirin in ischaemic cerebrovascular disease. How strong is the case for a different dosing regimen? *Stroke.* **27**: 756–60.

Robertson N, Baker R and Hearnshaw H (1996) Changing the clinical behaviour of doctors – a psychological framework. *Quality in Health Care.* **5**: 51–4.

Royal College of General Practitioners (1995) *The Development and Implementation of Clinical Guidelines.* Report from practice 26. RCGP, London.

Sackett D L, Richardson W S, Rosenberg W and Haynes R B (1997) *Evidence-based Medicine: How to Practice and Teach EBM.* Churchill Livingstone, London.

Secretaries of State for Health, Social Services, Wales, Northern Ireland and Scotland (1989) *Working for Patients.* CMN 555. HMSO, London.

Soumerai S B and Avorn J (1990) Principles of educational outreach ('academic detailing') to improve clinical decision making. *Journal of the American Medical Association.* **263**: 549–56.

Soumerai S B, Salem-Schatz S, Avorn J *et al.* (1993) A controlled trial of educational outreach to improve blood transfusion practice. *Journal of the American Medical Association.* **270**: 961–6.

van der Heijden G J M G, van der Windt D A W M, Kleijnen J *et al.* (1996) Steroid injections for shoulder disorders: a systematic review of randomized clinical trials. *British Journal of General Practice.* **46**: 309–16.

Wayne A R, Blazer D G, Schaffner W *et al.* (1986) Reducing long-term diazepam prescribing in office practice. *Journal of the American Medical Association.* **256**: 2536–9.

Wensing M and Grol R (1994) Single and combined strategies for implementing changes in primary care: a literature review. *International Journal for Quality in Health Care.* **6**: 115–32.

Yano E M, Fink A, Hirsch S H *et al.* (1995). Helping practices reach primary care goals. Lessons from the literature. *Archives of Internal Medicine.* **155**: 1146–59.

Zikmund W G and d'Amico M (1996) *Basic Marketing.* West Publishing Company, Minneapolis.

# Further reading

Dunn E V, Norton P G, Stewart M *et al.* (eds) (1994) *Disseminating Research/Changing Practice.* Sage Publications, Thousand Oaks.

Royal College of General Practitioners (1995) *The Development and Implementation of Clinical Guidelines.* Report from practice 26. RCGP, London.

Sackett D L, Richardson W S, Rosenberg W and Haynes R B (1997) *Evidence-based Medicine: How to Practice and Teach EBM.* Churchill Livingstone, London.

# Glossary

**Abstract**     a very concise overview of an article.

**Abstracting journals**     contain lists of references to journal articles, each one listed with the abstract. Lists are arranged under subject headings.

**Anonymity**     is the protection of the identity of research subjects such that even the researcher cannot identify the respondent to a questionnaire. Questionnaires in an anonymous survey do not have an identification number and cannot be linked back to an individual. Anonymity should not be confused with confidentiality where individuals can be identified by the researcher.

**Audit**     the systematic critical analysis of the quality of medical care, including the procedures used for diagnosis and treatment, the use of resources and the resulting outcome and quality of life for the patient.

**Beneficence**     is the principle of furthering the legitimate interests of others.

**Bias**     is a deviation of the results from the truth. This can either be due to random error or, more likely, systematic error. The latter could be caused by, for example, sampling or poor questionnaire design.

**Bibliographic tools**     indexing or abstracting journals to help locate literature.

**Blind study**     is one in which subjects in an experiment do not know which treatment they are to receive, i.e. the real intervention or the placebo. Blind studies are commonly undertaken in drug trials because the placebo effect is so great that it can radically alter outcome measures. In a blind study only the patient does not know which intervention he/she is receiving. The researcher administering the intervention does know. See 'double blind' and 'triple blind'.

**Case–control study**     an observational epidemiologic study comparing a group of people with a disease (cases) with a group of people without the disease (controls) in terms of exposure to a risk factor. The groups should be similar in terms of certain characteristics (such as age and sex).

**CD-ROM**

compact disc read by computers. Used to store references to the literature.

**Clinical practice guidelines**

systematically developed statements to assist practitioner and patient decisions about appropriate healthcare for specific clinical circumstances.

**Cohort study**

a prospective epidemiologic study that takes a defined population which experiences different degrees of exposure to a risk factor and is observed over time to compare incidence rates across different exposure levels.

**Confidentiality**

is the protection of the identity of research subjects so that identities cannot be revealed in the research findings and the only person who can link a respondent's completed questionnaire to a name and address is the researcher. A questionnaire with just a coded identification number is confidential. This should not be confused with anonymity where not even the researcher can identify the subjects.

**Constant error**

can be caused by the presence of a confounding variable in an experiment. It is also an alternative term for systematic bias.

**Construct validity**

is the extent to which measurement corresponds to the theoretical concepts (constructs) concerning the object of the study. There are two kinds of construct validity: convergent and divergent.

**Content validity**

is a set of operations or measures which together operationalise all aspects of a concept.

**Control group**

is the group in an experiment that is not exposed to the intervention or independent variable. The control group exists to provide a baseline comparison for the intervention group so as to measure the influence of the independent variable.

**Criterion validity**

is the extent to which measurement correlates with an external indicator of the phenomenon. There are two types of criterion validity: concurrent and predictive – (i) concurrent validity is a comparison against another external measurement at the same point in time; (ii) predictive validity is the extent to which the measurement can act as a predictor of the criterion. Predictive validity can be useful in relation to health since it can act as an early risk indicator before a condition develops in full.

| | |
|---|---|
| **Cross-sectional survey** | a study design that takes a 'snap shot' of the population at a particular moment in time. It is not longitudinal and subjects are not followed up. |
| **Deontological** | is derived from the Greek 'deon' meaning duty. |
| **Dissemination** | the distribution of information relating to the study (particularly its findings) to groups, agencies and organisations who are potentially affected by the findings. |
| **Double blind** | is a procedure in which neither the subjects nor the researcher know which treatment the subject has been assigned to, i.e. either the real intervention or the placebo. This format is commonly used in drug trials to prevent biasing the outcome. See 'blind study' and 'triple blind'. |
| **Eligibility criteria** | are an agreed set of characteristics that patients or subjects need to satisfy before they can be included or sampled for inclusion into the study. These may include age range, gender, presentation to a certain service, receiving specific treatment, registration with a practice or a combination of factors. |
| **Error** | can be due to two sources: random error and systematic error. Random error is due to chance, whilst systematic error is due to an identifiable source such as sampling bias or response bias. |
| **Evaluation** | a systematic investigation into the effectiveness of a service or intervention according to agreed objectives. |
| **Exposure** | a risk or protective factor shared by some or all of a study group, for example smoking, family history of heart disease or vitamin supplements. |
| **External validity** | relates to the extent to which the findings from a study can be generalised (from the sample) to a wider population (and be claimed to be representative). |
| **Face validity** | is the extent that the measure or instrument being used appears to measure what it is supposed to. For example, a thermometer might be said to possess face validity. |
| **Flesch Reading Ease Score** | computes readability based on the average number of syllables per word and the average number of words per sentence. Scores range from 0 (zero) to 100. Standard writing usually scores between 60 and 70. The higher the score, the greater the number of people who can easily |

understand the document. This is available as a facility under Word for Windows.

**Fog Index**            calculates the reading age of written material using the following steps:

(1) Select a sample of at least 100 words.
(2) Divide the total number of words in the extract by the number of sentences. This gives the average length of sentence.
(3) Count the number of words with three or more syllables. This is the number of 'hard words'.
(4) Add the number of hard words to the average number of words in a sentence. Multiply this figure by 0.4. The answer corresponds to the years of education needed to easily understand this piece of writing. A score of 18 plus represents a college graduate. Bear in mind that the reading age of *The Sun* newspaper is around 12.

**Generalisability**      the extent to which findings can be extended from the study sample to the wider population the sample represents.

**Grant-holder**       one of the named applicants on a successful grant application responsible for carrying out the funded research.

**Grant-making body**    organisation or agency who award research grants.

**Indexing journals**     contain lists of references to journal articles. Lists are arranged under subject headings.

**Informed consent**    is the term associated with research of human subjects and is concerned with the extent to which prospective participants are made aware of the exact nature of the research and their right to agree or decline to participate.

**Instrument validity**    is the extent to which the instrument or indicator measures what it purports to measure. Note that a study could have instrument validity but still lack validity overall due to lack of external validity.

**Internal validity**     relates to the validity of the study itself, including both the design and the instruments used.

**Intervention**        is related to the independent variable in an experimental design. An intervention could take the form of treatment, such as a drug treatment. Those subjects selected to receive the intervention in an experiment are placed in the 'intervention' group.

**Interview**  a method of data collection which may range from structured (where questions and a permissible range of answers are predetermined) to unstructured (where neither the questions nor the form of answers are set out in advance).

**Journals**  magazine-sized publications containing articles.

**Justice**  is the principle of being fair to all concerned.

**Keywords**  words or terms used to categorise and identify published research papers.

**Literature**  all published written work.

**Literature reviews**  a concise summary of published work on a specified subject.

**Monograph**  an in-depth report on a specified subject published in book format.

**On-line**  a connection via a computer network to a large remote computer that holds references to the literature.

**Outcome measure**  a measure of an aspect of health considered to be potentially affected by an intervention that has taken place.

**Piloting**  the process of testing out any aspect of a study design.

**Placebo**  is usually an inert drug or 'sugar-coated pill' used to simulate drug treatment in a control group in an experimental design. Placebo is Latin for 'I will please'.

**Power**  statistical power is the measure of the extent to which a study is capable of discerning significant differences or associations that exist within the population under investigation, and is of critical importance whenever a hypothesis is tested by statistics. Conventionally, studies should reach a power level of 0.8, such that four times out of five a null hypothesis will be rejected by a study. Statistical power may be most easily increased by increasing the sample size.

**Prevalence**  the number of cases of a certain condition in a specific population at a designated time.

**Process measure**  an indication of the level of service provision and uptake (for example number of patients attending health promotion clinics, or ratio of home visits to surgery visits).

| | |
|---|---|
| **Proposal** | a plan of investigation, including background of study, study protocol and full costing. |
| **Protocol** | a detailed step-by-step plan to be followed during the period of study. |
| **Qualitative research** | deals with the human experience and is based on the analysis of words rather than numbers. Qualitative research methods seek to explore rich information usually collected from fairly small samples and include methods such as in-depth interviews, focus groups, action research and ethnographic studies. |
| **Quantitative research** | is essentially concerned with numerical measurement and numerical data. All experimental research is based on a quantitative approach. Quantitative research tends to be based on larger sample sizes in order to produce results that can be generalised to a wider population. |
| **Questionnaire** | is a set of questions used to collect data. Questionnaires can be administered face to face by an interviewer, over a telephone or by self-completion. Questionnaires can include closed or open-ended questions. |
| **Randomisation** | is the process by which subjects are assigned to groups (for example, experimental or control) to avoid investigator bias. The method is predetermined using tables of random numbers or computer-generated random assignment. |
| **Randomised controlled trial (RCT)** | an experiment in which subjects are randomly allocated to groups (sometimes referred to as 'arms'). These groups are usually experimental (receiving a specific intervention) and control (not receiving the intervention). The two groups are then compared in terms of the outcome measure of the study. |
| **Recruits** | subjects who agree to take part in a study. Usually used in the context of experimental research. |
| **Referee** | expert reviewer of a grant application. |
| **Reliability** | is concerned with the extent to which a measure gives consistent results. It is also a precondition for validity. |
| **Representativeness** | is the extent to which a sample of subjects is representative of the wider population. If a sample is not representative then the findings may not be generalisable. |

**Response rate**          the number of respondents who agree to participate in a study divided by the number of respondents invited to participate and expressed as a percentage.

**Review criteria**        systematically developed statements that can be used to assess the appropriateness of specific healthcare decisions, services and outcomes.

**Sampling frame**         a list of the sampling units used in the selection of the sample. Examples of sampling frames are local electoral rolls and practice registers.

**Systematic review**      a scientifically rigorous review of research literature that follows explicit steps for the identification and inclusion of studies, and for combing the evidence from the studies.

**Triple blind**           a procedure in which not only are the subjects and the researcher administering the intervention blinded but also the person carrying out the data analysis. The data are coded so that it is not possible for the analyst to identify which is the intervention group and which is the control group in order to prevent bias.

**Validity**               is the extent to which a study measures what it purports to measure. There are many different types of validity.

# Index